Why Conscience Matters

The book provides a detailed introduction to a major debate in bioethics and a rigorous account of the role of conscience in professional decision-making.

Exploring the role of conscience in healthcare practice, this book offers fresh counterpoints to recent calls to ban or severely restrict conscience objection. It provides a detailed philosophical account of the nature and moral import of conscience and defends a prima facie right to conscientious objection for healthcare professionals. The book also has relevance to broader debates about religious liberty and civil rights, such as debates about the rights and duties of persons and institutions who refuse services to clients on the basis of a religious objection. The book concludes with a discussion of how to regulate individual and institutional conscientious objection and presents general principles for the accommodation of individual conscientious objectors in the healthcare system.

This book will be of value to students and scholars in the fields of moral philosophy, bioethics and health law.

Xavier Symons is Postdoctoral Research Fellow, Plunket Centre for Ethics, Australian Catholic University and St Vincent's Health Australia. His research interests include ethical issues at the beginning and end of life, the ethics of healthcare resource allocation, and the ethics of conscientious objection. His work has been published in leading bioethics journals, and he is a regular contributor to the Australian media.

T0372896

Routledge Research in Applied Ethics

For more information about this series, please visit: www.routledge.com/Routledge-Research-in-Applied-Ethics/book-series/RRAES

Why Conscience Matters

A Defence of Conscientious Objection in Healthcare

Xavier Symons

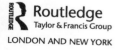 Routledge
Taylor & Francis Group

LONDON AND NEW YORK

First published 2023
by Routledge
4 Park Square, Milton Park, Abingdon, Oxon OX14 4RN

and by Routledge
605 Third Avenue, New York, NY 10158

Routledge is an imprint of the Taylor & Francis Group, an informa business

British Library Cataloguing-in-Publication Data
A catalogue record for this book is available from the British Library

Library of Congress Cataloging-in-Publication Data
A catalog record for this book has been requested

ISBN: 978-1-032-16226-3 (hbk)
ISBN: 978-1-032-16225-6 (pbk)
ISBN: 978-1-003-24762-3 (ebk)

DOI: 10.4324/9781003247623

Typeset in Times New Roman
by Apex CoVantage, LLC

Contents

Figures

Foreword

Conscience matters, but is the controversy really about conscience?

"Thus conscience doth make cowards of us all."
Shakespeare, *Hamlet*. Act 3, scene 1, line 83

The conscience of the medical practitioner has recently become a subject of intense ethical controversy. This would strike anyone not living in the 21st-century-Western academic world as exceedingly odd. Shouldn't everyone want physicians, nurses, pharmacists and other healthcare professionals to be people who act conscientiously? What could be controversial about that?

Ironically, the issue may just be that conscience is not the issue. The burning normative question is what to do when physicians or other healthcare professionals have moral objections to what patients ask them to do. As Xavier Symons demonstrates in this important new book, if one examines the question from the perspective of philosophical moral psychology and asks what conscience is and what role it ought to play in the life of a healthcare professional, no reasonable person can say that physicians ought to violate their consciences in order to practise medicine. As Symons notes, that would be an endorsement of a programme of systematic moral injury. Moreover, casting conscience as an idiosyncratic preference that can be suppressed (like a preference for pistachio ice cream) in order to meet the preferences of one's client is a mis-construal of what conscience is and what it means to be a moral agent in general and what it means to be a healthcare professional in particular.

I would argue, however, that even though the normative issue at stake is connected to questions about conscience, the fundamental problem is not about the limits of conscience or controversies about what conscience is. Rather, the problem resides in the realm of political philosophy and concerns two different questions: (1) what is the nature of a profession and its role in a pluralistic democratic republic? and (2) what does tolerance mean when it is applied to public practices that are morally controversial?

The word "conscience" has become affixed to questions about whether medical professionals can decline to perform acts that patients request, based on judgement that the requested act is immoral. This appears to have happened through the repeated use of the term "conscientious objection" in relationship to these medical controversies. The term "conscientious objection" has traditionally been used to describe a complex legal system by which an individual citizen with a relatively uncommon moral or religious conviction can be released from performing an almost universally recognised legal duty. Thus, for example, some individuals can be excused from taking an oath to tell the truth in court by claiming a conscientious objection to swearing. Up until the Vietnam War, the same was true of those who asked to be excused from the duty serve in the military – Quakers and other pacifists applied for (and often were granted) "conscientious objector" status. With the Vietnam conflict, however, moral opposition to the war became widespread, pacifism became more popular, and moral objection to the war, in some circles of discourse, soon became elided with conscientious objection. At around the same time, moral controversy over abortion was dividing the country and, in the wake of the U.S. Supreme Court's famous Roe v Wade decision legalising abortion, the U.S. Congress enacted legislation assuring that no practitioner with a moral objection to the controversial procedure would be required to participate in abortion. This assurance, passed with overwhelming bipartisan support (the vote was 92–1), was dubbed a "conscience clause", presumably because those who objected to abortion were understood to do so on moral grounds, just as the pacifist who objected to military service. Subsequently, practitioners who objected to participation in abortion began claiming that they were "conscientious objectors". As more moral controversial procedures have been introduced into medical care, those who refuse to participate have likewise called themselves "conscientious objectors" and are referred to as such by the press, legal scholars and bioethicists. Thus, the muddle we are in. Presumably anyone who holds any practice to be immoral would be acting contrary to conscience by participating in that practice. Now, however, anyone who objects ethically to any practice can be called a conscientious objector. I, for one, am a conscientious objector to adultery, theft, tax evasion, and the torture of human beings, cats and other animals. The phrase has lost its linguistic bearings.

Casting the issue as one of "conscientious objection" also begs the ethical question because the idea of conscientious objection assumes that the default action is a widely recognised and long-standing duty from which one is asking to be granted an exception, rather than a deeply controversial and new practice. Calling these issues "conscientious objection" leads to discussions that frame the question at hand as one that pits physicians' rights to hold idiosyncratic religious beliefs against patients' rights to access necessary medical care that is universally held to be the duty of physicians to provide. The practices at issue, however, are deeply morally controversial, and the framework for ethical analysis cannot assume that the default position is that there is a moral duty to provide them. Talking in such terms miscasts the ethical issue by begging the question of the moral propriety of the ethically controversial practice.

Although he does not appear to object to the use of "conscientious objection", Symons is keenly aware of the various levels of ethical discourse at play when thinking about whether a just, tolerant, pluralistic, democratic republic ought to require medical practitioners to participate in medical procedures that they judge to be immoral. Specifically, the question at hand is this: When a morally controversial medical practice (X) is deemed legally permissible by a society in order to accommodate the moral beliefs of those who support X, does this entail a moral duty for each medical professional (M) in that society either to perform X upon the request of patient P or to assure that someone else performs X in order to satisfy the request from P, given medical conditions that supporters of X would deem safe, effective, and other things being equal, medically indicated, even if M believes that X is morally wrong? Call this the Central Question.

Symons, refreshingly, grounds his account of conscience and healthcare practice in philosophical moral psychology. He and I share the view that far too many authors commenting on the topic ignore this deeper groundwork, rendering their analyses shaky and their conclusions either weakly justified or flat out wrong. Symons adopts a form of what he calls an integrity view of conscience – a commitment to have and hold self-identifying moral commitments and to act in accord with those commitments such that failure to do so would be unthinkable to the person. He connects his account of conscience to the notion of seeing oneself as a moral agent and to the notion of virtue. Perhaps the most novel contribution he makes is by helping readers to understand that seeing oneself as a medical professional necessarily involves a conscientious commitment to practise according to a self-identifying set of moral principles and to grow in virtue so as to become the best physician, nurse, psychologist or other healthcare professional that one can be. This process requires a community of persons with a similar conscientious commitment and enough lived experience to have grown in those virtues themselves and enough insight to know how to pass them on to the next generation. Thus, only experienced professionals, ultimately, can train a new member of any given profession.

In considering the Central Question, Symons looks at the importance of being a member of a profession. He critically evaluates conceptions of the physician that are at odds with the notion of a professional, such as the "provider of services" model, or the notion of the physician as an agent of the state or a pure fiduciary model in which the task of the physician is always to advance the values of the patient. He concludes that none are adequate conceptions of a professional, and to the extent that these models underlie arguments that M must provide X to P, those arguments are unsound because they rely upon faulty understandings of what it means to be a professional. Symons is spot on here. A provider of goods and services, like a shoe salesman, will sell a customer shoes even if they are ugly and ill-fitting, so long as the patient seems to like them. Physicians, by contrast, are obliged to refrain from providing what they think will not heal a patient, even if it is desired by the patient. Nor should physicians be seen as agents of the state. History is rife with examples of medicine being co-opted by the state to do all sorts of immoral things, like assisting in torture or declaring political dissidents mentally ill. Nor is a physician a pure fiduciary of the patient. Public health concerns, for example, can limit what a physician does for a patient, and the ideal is a model in which the patient and the physician undertake a joint enterprise aiming at a common goal – making (or keeping) the patient well.

As Symons argues, medical acts, as professional acts, are both technical and moral. This requires that clinicians always be granted a very wide latitude in the judgements they make. These judgements require the virtues to which I alluded earlier, including practical wisdom, compassion and fidelity, all informed by a judgement about what is best for the patient. To eradicate the element of moral judgement from medical practice is to undermine what medicine must do in order to function as a profession.

Symons does not comment at length on the political philosophy of the Central Question, but I think there are two aspects that impact upon how society responds to that question. The first political philosophical observation I would make is that a healthy, pluralistic, liberal, democratic republic needs strong institutions that are distinct from the state and the market in order to balance power and to function well. Among these institutions are the academy, religions and the professions. Professions must not be instruments of either the market or the state, and one of the problems with the models of the physician's role that Symons criticises is that they tie the profession too closely to either the market or the state, creating unhealthy imbalances in power.

The second political question is that of tolerance, which is the category under which questions like the Central Question are best addressed. If X is made legal in the face of intense disagreement within society about whether it is morally appropriate, majorities should not force minorities to participate in X. If X is a controversial medical procedure that society has decided should be legally permissible, patients should be free to pursue X and find physicians who will perform or provide X, but it is an instance of the tyranny of the majority to force all physicians (M) to provide X. While the physician who objects morally to X presumably does so conscientiously, the issue ought not to be understood as one of conscientious objection as in the case of the conscription of a committed pacifist but as one of tolerance in a healthy pluralistic, liberal, democratic republic. A healthy pluralistic, liberal, democratic republic not only tolerates intellectual dissent from ethically controversial practices but also, a fortiori, refrains from forcing dissenters to perform those practices.

While he does not engage the Central Question at the level of political philosophy, Symons does provide a suggested political solution. While opponents of "the conscience rights" of healthcare professionals have suggested that those with a moral objection who will not provide a legal medical service ought to advertise their objections, Symons suggests the opposite – those who will provide the service should make it clear and publicly known that they will. He proposes a searchable database of those who will provide the service. This makes immense sense. It is how things are usually done in other, non-controversial areas of medicine. For example, I am certified as a U.S. Civil Surgeon and perform immigration exams. There is a database of U.S. Civil Surgeons that can be searched for those who need a medical exam in order to change their immigration status. Since the vast majority of physicians are not certified as U.S. Civil Surgeons, this system makes much more sense than publishing a database of those who are not and asking patents to perform the onerous task of deducing that a particular physician will be able to perform an immigration exam by determining that they are not on the list of those who aren't. Likewise, the vast majority of U.S. physicians, even the vast majority of obstetrician-gynaecologists, do not perform abortions. It would be of more practical help to patients seeking an abortion to find a list of those who will perform the procedure than to try to find a physician who is not on the list of those who won't.

Symons also argues for protecting the rights of institutions with particular moral commitments to opt out of morally controversial medical interventions. He disagrees with me that institutions can be said to have consciences, largely because he argues that institutions are incapable of experiencing the emotional sanction of violations of their fundamental moral commitments – what are often referred to as the "pangs" of conscience. This turns on how important those feelings are to the notion of conscience and whether conscience is some sort of mental faculty. It is true that an institution does not have a mind and does not experience emotions qua institution. Yet institutions do have fundamental moral commitments and hold themselves accountable to their fundamental commitments, just as individuals do. Institutions commonly enshrine these commitments in statements of mission, vision and values. Individual members of the institution may experience emotional discomfort if the institution fails to meet those commitments even if the institution, qua institution, does not. Such emotional reactions or rational assessments by individual members of an institution regarding whether a practice is consistent with the institution's fundamental commitments will undoubtedly impact the judgements made by those who act on behalf of the institution. We could quibble about whether that is sufficient to enable us to say that there is such a thing as institutional conscience. Nonetheless, Symons agrees that the combination of these institutional commitments and the capacity of institutions for collective action are enough to allow us to say that Central Question should be answered for institutions just as it should be for individuals – we ought to respect the rights of institutions to opt out of medical acts that violate their self-identifying moral commitments. Accordingly, Symons and I have no disagreement about the ethical evaluation of the matter. And if I am right that the real issues at stake are tolerance and pluralism rather than conscience, then whether one calls the collective commitments and judgements of institutions "conscience" does not matter. What matters is that a healthy pluralistic, liberal, democratic republic recognises the value of institutions with fundamental moral commitments and tolerates institutions that will not perform morally controversial acts that the society as a whole deems morally permissible. True pluralism recognises and respects a diversity of institutions and a diversity of individuals, in their fundamental moral commitments and in their identities.

Symons has made an important contribution to the debate on how to resolve disagreements regarding the provision of morally controversial but legally permissible medical interventions. This book is clear, careful, philosophically sound, insightful and practical all at once. While it is unlikely to be persuasive to all, no one concerned about these issues will be able to ignore it.

Daniel P. Sulmasy, MD, PhD
Washington, DC
January 12, 2022

Preface

This book is the fruit of several years of reflection on the topic of conscientious objection. I began writing about conscientious objection in healthcare almost a decade ago while working for the online bioethics news service BioEdge. Conscientious objection was beginning to generate a stir in the academic literature, and complex questions were arising in different jurisdictions debating legislation concerning elective abortion and voluntary euthanasia. The first example to catch my attention was the Abortion Act 2008 (VIC) – a highly controversial piece of legislation enacted in the Australian state of Victoria. Section 8 of the Abortion Act obliged registered medical practitioners with a conscientious objection to refer patients seeking an abortion to "another registered health practitioner in the same regulated health profession who . . . does not have a conscientious objection to abortion". The legislation also declared that registered medical practitioners are "under a duty to perform an abortion in an emergency where the abortion is necessary to preserve the life of the pregnant woman". The public debate surrounding the Abortion Act was intense and polemical, though it seems like the issue of conscientious objection in healthcare has only become more neuralgic in the years since the passage of this law.

This book is also inspired by a series of classroom debates on conscientious objection that I had with Professor Julian Savulescu at the University of Melbourne Law School. The debates were part of a medical ethics course that Julian taught in the Law School's Masters of Law programme. Julian invited me – an academic working within the Catholic ethical tradition – to make the case "in favour" of conscientious objection in healthcare. In these debates, I shared with students a vision of conscientious objection in medicine that characterised judgements of conscience as the fruit of humble and considered moral reflection on one's professional experience. Judgements of conscience in clinical medicine do not entail moral or epistemic arrogance. On the contrary, they are the product of a moral journey that all clinicians undergo as they seek to identify how to realise the goods of medicine in different clinical situations. This seemed to resonate with the audience, which was a mix of clinicians and laypeople. The idea that we form our consciences by virtue of reflection on experience and through guidance from peers cohered with the audience's intuitions about moral formation. This has led me to believe that there is something intuitively plausible about respect for conscience in healthcare practice.

There is a strong policy dimension to this book, and it is my hope that it will be of some assistance to readers involved in health policy. Abortion and euthanasia legislation is one obvious area of relevance. Yet the COVID-19 pandemic has also highlighted the importance of thinking about conscientious objection in the context of public health and, specifically, the practice of conscientious objection to vaccination. Vaccine mandates have been introduced in jurisdictions around the world which limit the ability of doctors and other healthcare professionals to object to receiving vaccines. This has provided a useful counterpoint to the beginning and end-of-life issues that typically serve as the focus for conscientious objection. I will not deal directly with the ethics of medical conscientious objection to vaccination, but I hope that the framework outlined in this book will assist policymakers in thinking through relevant issues.

This book is also intended to help moral philosophers think more deeply about questions pertaining to conscience. Conscience presupposes a personal engagement with morality; and yet conscience has been largely overlooked in the history of modern moral philosophy. It is my hope that this book will contribute in a modest way to moral philosophical scholarship on conscience by providing a detailed account of how conscience relates to questions of meaning and purpose in the lives of moral agents. One wonders whether moral philosophy is failing in one of its most important tasks if we fail to think deeply about what it means to form one's moral character and acquire a sense of meaning and purpose in life.

Finally, we ought to recognise how the issue of conscientious objection comes apart from questions pertaining to the morality of abortion, euthanasia and socially contentious services provided by medical practitioners today. In our polarised society, it is often difficult for people to see how one bioethical commitment – say, support for abortion – need not entail other bioethical commitments such as support for a ban on conscientious objection to abortion. But we should recognise that these are two very different issues. First-order debates about the morality of abortion and euthanasia and second-order debates about the morality of conscientious objection require a consideration of a whole different set of moral arguments. One of the reasons why the conscientious objection debate might seem to be at an impasse is that scholars often regress back to a debate about the morality or immorality of particular procedures rather than bracketing off these questions to deal with the separate question of whether practitioners should be allowed to opt out of providing these procedures. This book aims to show how the case for conscientious objection can be made independent of first-order debates about the morality of medical procedures.

I offer this book in the spirit of charitable academic exchange and in a spirit of friendship. I have not taken an ideological approach to this material, which is so often a temptation. It is my hope that this book will stimulate interest in conscience and also a desire to better understand the link between conscience and conscientious objection.

Georgetown University
December 2021

Acknowledgements

This book has been a long time in gestation, and I ought to thank several people for their support at various stages of the writing process. First, I would like to thank those who were most directly involved in the drafting of this manuscript. This includes Mark Murphy and James Franklin, who provided detailed feedback on earlier drafts of the manuscript, as well as Bernadette Tobin, Michal Pruski, Paul Hanna, Daniel Rodger and Grace Yeung, who all read draft chapters.

Several others played an important role in the conception of this book. I would like to thank Roger Crisp for encouraging me to write a book after attending a seminar paper that I delivered at the Uehiro Centre in Oxford in December 2019. I would also like to thank Julian Savulescu for the opportunity to join his Melbourne University law classes over the past few years and engage in fruitful discussions with students about conscientious objection in medicine. A thank you is also in order for Dr Chris French for pressing me to investigate the relationship between conscience and conscientious objection.

I would like to thank my mentors – Bernadette Tobin, Margaret Somerville and Christian Miller – for their extensive career advice. I am immensely grateful to Daniel P. Sulmasy for his generous comments in the foreword of this book.

Lastly, I would like to thank Michael Cook for his general advice and support, and guidance over the years, starting with my employment at BioEdge. Michael's deep bioethical insight is only surpassed in excellence by his generosity in offering feedback on hastily written drafts.

1   Introduction

Conscience revisited

Introduction

Conscience is an idea that has significant currency in everyday language. We regularly hear of people "searching their conscience" or being guided by the "inner voice of conscience". Someone who acts with an upright intention is said to act "in good conscience" while someone who feels moral regret is said to have a "guilty conscience". Conscience also features in political discourse – from "conscience votes" in parliaments to "prisoners of conscience" imprisoned on account of their political or religious beliefs. Few scholars, however, acknowledge the connection between conscience and conscientious objection in healthcare. There is, in fact, increasing scepticism towards appeals to conscience that underpin practitioners' conscientious objections. Many theorists see conscience as a realm of personal opinion that cannot possibly serve as a basis for moral decision-making in medicine.

Indeed, an anomalous feature of contemporary bioethics literature is its aggressively critical view of the practice of conscientious objection. Many ethicists argue that the practice of accommodating conscientious objection in healthcare interferes with the primary duty of healthcare professionals to promote patient welfare (Savulescu 2006; Savulescu and Schuklenk 2017; Stahl and Emanuel 2017). That is, the practice of conscientious objection is said to impede timely access to medical care for patients or may result in harm to their health (Strickland 2012; Schuklenk and Smalling 2017; Schuklenk 2018; Keogh *et al.* 2019). In light of this, a consensus has emerged in some academic circles that conscientious objection should be heavily restricted if allowed at all.

This book seeks to challenge such a consensus. The subsequent chapters develop a detailed account of conscience with the aim of defending the exercise of conscience in medicine, which necessarily includes the practice of conscientious objection. I seek to answer the fundamental question of why conscience is important and why it is costly for clinicians to act contrary to their conscience. I will argue that freedom of conscience is of paramount importance, inseparable from medical practice, and that restricting a medical professional's right to conscientious objection can have a harmful impact on individual agents as well as the practice of healthcare. Conscience is fundamental to moral judgement, and it

DOI: 10.4324/9781003247623-1

is a means by which medical practitioners navigate the ethical complexities that characterise their everyday work. Restricting physicians' conscience rights paradoxically stunts their acquisition of professional virtue and limits their capacity for independent practical reasoning. This has significant implications not just for individual medical practitioners but for the profession in general.

In providing a detailed account of conscience, this book seeks in a modest way to stimulate scholarly interest in conscience and the implications that conscience might have for our understanding of ethics in medical practice. It is regrettable that recent moral philosophical scholarship in the anglophone world is characterised by a dearth of research on the topic of conscience and its relevance to professional life. This manuscript seeks to encourage further research on the relevance of conscience to professional ethics.

In this introductory chapter, I will situate the argument of this book within its academic, social and political context. Section 1 offers an account of the meaning of conscience as it is employed in this book, while Section 2 offers a definition of the term "conscientious objector". In Section 3, I discuss the practice of conscientious objection in healthcare today. In Section 4, I briefly discuss the state of the academic literature on conscientious objection and offer an overview of the central thesis of this book. Section 5 makes some brief clarificatory remarks on the argumentative strategy employed in this book, while Section 6 offers a precis of the subsequent chapters.

1. The meaning of conscience

The term 'conscience' can be used in several ways, and it is important to be clear on the sense in which I am using the word 'conscience' in this book. The following list identifies several operations that are commonly said to be the work of conscience. Conscience is said to be responsible for the following:

1   Immediate moral judgements on particular cases (i.e. that an agent ought to "do this" and "avoid that") (Rousseau 1762/1921; Butler 1726/1950). For example, we might think of an adolescent's judgement that stealing a candy bar from the local convenience store is an act of theft and ought not to be pursued. This could be said to be an instance in which conscience is at work in the moral psychology of the adolescent agent.
2   Judgements about basic moral principles of morality. We might, for example, think of the foundational judgement that many if not most moral agents reach about the moral equality of persons. Such a judgement forms the basis of one's conception of morality, and one might argue that these foundational judgements are the work of conscience.
3   The cognitive judgement that good is to be followed and evil avoided. This is perhaps the most basic moral judgement that an agent can make, and, indeed, it is arguably presupposed in all moral reasoning that humans engage in. The scholastics called this judgement *synderesis*, and some have translated this notion into English as "conscience" (Hoffmann 2012).

4 A commitment to acting in accord with what one knows to be right and good. It is not enough for moral agents to know the good; one must have a desire to actually do it. Some moral theorists (Fuss 1964; Sulmasy 2008) have argued that conscience is principally concerned with an existential commitment to living in accord with one's own considered understanding of morality.

The sense in which I use conscience in this book is closest to point 4, though even that does not capture the full role that I attribute to conscience. Conscience, in my view, has two interrelated functions. It involves a commitment to know and understand morality and also a commitment to act with integrity. It involves a desire to know what is good and right and also a desire to act in accord with the moral principles that characterise one's moral outlook. Conscience, furthermore, shapes moral character. It leads agents to grapple deeply with the complexities of everyday moral life and to form considered moral views about the nature of morality and one's own moral responsibilities. These views, in turn, come to constitute part of one's character. Character formation, then, is one important function of conscience.

It is not my intention, however, to deny that conscience performs the other operations identified in points 1 to 3. On the contrary, I am sympathetic to accounts of conscience that suggest that it provides us with both general and particular moral knowledge. For the purposes of this book, however, I will bracket off this alternative view of conscience and will focus on conscience's role in preserving moral integrity and motivating agents to act in accord with their own considered understanding of morality. It is this sense of conscience that I believe is most relevant to debates about conscientious objection. Conscience is an important source of guidance to the morally perplexed; yet more fundamentally it is the feature of human psychology that leads a moral agent to desire to know morality and also to act in accord with one's moral responsibilities.

2. A definition of "conscientious objector"

Historically, the term "conscientious objector" was first applied to a group of citizens in late 19th-century England who refused vaccination for smallpox. The British Vaccination Act of 1898 provided a conscience clause to allow exemptions to mandatory smallpox vaccination, thus giving rise to the term "conscientious objector" that we use today (Wolfe and Sharpe 2002). The focus of this book, however, will be physicians rather than healthcare consumers. In the context of healthcare provision, conscientious objectors are practitioners or entities that opt out of the provision of a procedure or service due to a perceived normative conflict between the service and a practitioner's or entity's deeply held beliefs or commitments. An example of this would be a Catholic gynaecologist who has a moral objection to terminations of pregnancy and who refuses to provide an elective abortion for patients who request the service. Alternatively, we might think of a Christian hospice service that refuses to credential physicians wishing to provide assessments for euthanasia for residents on site. Conscientious objectors, however, need not be religious. The defining feature of a conscientious objector in medicine is that they opt out of the provision of a medical service because they believe that the service would be harmful to the welfare of the patient and/or in some way contrary to the goals of medicine.

To be clear, conscientious objectors do *not* act based on distaste for some aspect or other of one's professional work. Rather, their objections are based on a particular view of medicine and the morality of certain procedures or services that have been requested by patients. We ought, therefore, to distinguish what we might call sincere and authentic conscientious objections from a mere dislike of some aspect of one's job. Sometimes a doctor may choose not to provide a service to a patient simply because they find this service tiresome or distasteful. This should not be confused with a genuine appeal to conscience, in which a healthcare professional opts not to participate in the provision of a service on account of a moral objection. Authors may conflate these two very different phenomena, but they ought to be distinguished. In this book, I will take conscientious objection to refer to the refusal by healthcare professionals to participate in medical practices on the grounds of genuine, deeply held, reasonable ethical convictions about the proper goals of medicine and healthcare. I set to one-side cases where the objection is of a dubious character (such as where a clinician merely finds a practice distasteful or tiresome).

Conscientious objection in medicine is not confined to the small set of socially contentious procedures such as abortion, contraception and euthanasia that receive most attention in the bioethics literature (Callahan 2005). Indeed, most of healthcare is concerned with issues other than abortion, contraception and euthanasia. Medical practitioners are required to make complex judgements in a variety of areas about the ethical advisability of medical care. Consider a transplant specialist who is asked to perform a kidney transplant operation on an 80-year-old patient. The specialist may have an objection to the allocation of a scarce resource like an organ to an octogenarian patient; they may refuse to perform the transplant on this basis. The doctor in this case has made an ethical judgement that the provision of treatment is not an ethically permissible allocation of resources and so ought to be withheld from the patient (Savulescu and Schuklenk 2017, 165). Or consider a fertility specialist who is approached by a couple about performing gender-selective In Vitro Fertilization for non-medical reasons. The fertility specialist may be concerned about the sexist bias latent in the couple's reasons for wanting a male child; the specialist might politely inform the couple that she is unwilling to provide the requested procedure. The fertility specialist in this case has made an ethical judgement about the motivations of the patient requesting the service and has withheld the service on this basis (King 2007, 418). The circumstances in which a doctor may conscientiously object, then, are many and varied, and we should not confine our understanding of conscientious objection to a small subset of medical procedures. Rather, conscientious objection in healthcare could refer to any procedure that a clinician believes is not in accord with the proper aims of medicine.

An important corollary is that the exercise of conscience is a feature of medical practice as such and not just some particular facet of medicine. Conscientious objection, then, ought not to be held to be something foreign to medical practice but rather ought to be conceived of as a natural part of the exercise of clinical judgement in medicine. This is a central claim in the argument advanced in this book, namely that conscience ought not to be conceived as something extraneous to medical practice but rather should be seen as an indispensable feature of ordinary decision-making in medicine.

It is appropriate here – given the current global pandemic – to make mention of medical practitioners who refuse to receive and/or administer COVID-19 vaccines. A small subset of primary care doctors around the world have opted out of receiving and/or administering COVID-19 vaccines to patients on the basis of an objection to some aspect or other of COVID-19 vaccines or the vaccine roll-out. This has been the source of significant frustration for health authorities seeking to ensure that patients receive timely access to vaccines and are protected from serious COVID-19-related illness. Some physicians, however, argued that they ought to be recognised as conscientious objectors and ought to be permitted to opt out of administering or receiving the COVID-19 vaccine. Irish general practitioner Dr Gerard Waters, for example, unsuccessfully attempted to be officially recognised by the Irish Medical Council as a conscientious objector to COVID-19 vaccination, arguing that pathogenicity of COVID-19 was not sufficiently severe to justify the administration of a "hastily developed" vaccine.[1] Granted, it is not just primary care doctors who have objected to COVID-19 vaccination. Professor Aaron Kheriaty of the University of California Irvine (UCI), an American psychiatrist and medical ethicist, was fired from his academic and clinical roles at UCI for refusing to receive a COVID-19 vaccine. Kheriaty had already contracted COVID-19 by the time a university-wide staff vaccine mandate was introduced. He argued that natural immunity from COVID-19 was equal to or superior to vaccination for COVID-19. At the time of writing, Professor Kheriaty was suing the university for his dismissal (Kheriaty 2021).

I do not intend to provide a detailed exploration of the topic of conscientious objection to COVID-19 vaccination. Suffice to say here that the issue of conscientious objection to COVID-19 vaccination demonstrates that conscientious objection in medicine is not just concerned with abortion or euthanasia and that we should be careful about reducing debate to these issues alone. A moral right to conscientious objection may be invoked (licitly or illicitly) in any context in medicine. It is my hope that the discussion in this book will provide readers with a framework with which to think through the ethics of conscientious objection to vaccination as well as the ethics of conscientious objection to abortion, euthanasia and the myriad of other procedures that characterise contemporary healthcare.

As stated, the term "conscientious objector" does not only apply to individual medical practitioners. Healthcare institutions may also refuse to provide particular medical procedures and thus can be termed "conscientious objectors". A Catholic healthcare network, for example, may choose not to participate in the provision of euthanasia in a jurisdiction where euthanasia is legal. This issue has come to the fore in recent years with the introduction of euthanasia legislation in countries such as Canada and Australia where Catholic providers make up a significant portion of the health and aged-care sector (White *et al*. 2021; Kirby 2021). Lawmakers have been forced to confront the question of whether euthanasia legislation should mandate that all health and aged-care providers be obliged to facilitate access to euthanasia for eligible patients.

The notion of *institutional conscientious objection* has been heavily criticised in recent bioethics scholarship (Durland 2011; Nelson 2018; Barczak 2019). In the penultimate chapter of this book, I will offer an account of the nature of institutions and institutional conscientious objection and seek to respond to some common criticisms of institutional conscientious objection.

3. Conscientious objection in healthcare practice

In this section I will offer a series of real-world vignettes of conscientious objection in healthcare practice and will also consider how conscientious objection is regulated in law and in professional codes of conduct. This will illustrate the relevance and immediacy of discussions concerning the ethics of conscientious objection.

Recent examples of conscientious objection in healthcare

In some jurisdictions, healthcare professionals have a limited legal right to opt out of direct participation in procedures to which they have a moral or religious objection. Typically, this right is defined in reference to specific procedures rather than as a general right. The main piece of legislation governing abortion in the United Kingdom, for example, contains a provision specifying a limited right to conscientious objection for healthcare professionals. Section 4 of the Abortion Act 1967 (UK) states that

> no person shall be under any duty, whether by contract or by any statutory or other legal requirement, to participate in any treatment authorised by this Act to which he has a conscientious objection.

This provision has historically been defined as referring to *direct participation* in abortion, such as a nurse assisting a doctor in performing an abortion, rather than *remote participation* in abortion, such as a receptionist typing a referral for a patient to abortion clinic. Conscientious objection to the former is permissible under the act; conscientious objection to the latter is not (UK Supreme Court 2014).[2]

Similar conscientious objection provisions exist in the law governing euthanasia and assisted suicide in certain jurisdictions. The Australian state of Victoria, for example, affords individual healthcare professionals a broad right to conscientious objection to participation in euthanasia (or *voluntary assisted dying*, as it is called in Victorian legislation). Section 7 of the Voluntary Assisted Dying Act 2017 (Vic) states:

> A registered health practitioner who has a conscientious objection to voluntary assisted dying has the right to refuse to do any of the following – (a) to

provide information about voluntary assisted dying; (b) to participate in the request and assessment process; (c) to apply for a voluntary assisted dying permit; (d) to supply, prescribe or administer a voluntary assisted dying substance; (e) to be present at the time of administration of a voluntary assisted dying substance; (f) to dispense a prescription for a voluntary assisted dying substance.

In effect, Victorian euthanasia law allows healthcare professionals with a conscientious objection to opt out of participation in any part of the process of its voluntary assisted dying regime (Victorian Government 2017). This conscientious objection clause is significantly broader than that found in The Abortion Act 2008 (VIC), which requires objecting doctors to refer their patients to a suitable practitioner willing to perform the procedure requested.

There are, however, jurisdictions in which doctors have no right to conscientiously object to participation in abortion or euthanasia. In Sweden, for example, there is no legal right to conscientious objection in healthcare. Conscientious objection, rather, is regulated under the country's labour laws. As Munthe (2017, 257) writes,

> Employees' requests to change work tasks are handled on a case-by-case basis within the frames of labour law, ensuring full voluntariness, and also employer's privilege regarding the organisation and direction of work, and duties of public institutions to provide services.

Healthcare providers have the power to impose penalties or dismiss employees who disrupt the provision of services that they (the provider) have deemed it appropriate to provide. An employee has no legal basis for demanding that their employer respect his or her conscientious objection.

These laws were put to the test in 2013 and 2014 when a Swedish midwife, Ellinor Grimmark, was denied employment by three separate health clinics in Sweden after she explained that she could not perform abortions due to her Christian faith. In Sweden, midwives are essentially nurses who specialise in pregnancy and child birth and seldom do abortions. The fact that Grimmark was a conscientious objector, however, appears to have been a source of concern for her potential employers. Grimmark took her would-be employers to court, arguing that she had been the subject of unfair discrimination. Her legal challenge was unsuccessful. The Swedish Appeals Court found that government health services can require healthcare professionals to perform and cooperate in abortions. Grimmark also appealed to the European Court of Human Rights (ECHR), but the ECHR found that Swedish authorities had acted lawfully in rescinding Grimmark's employment contracts.[3]

Most recent legal disputes about conscientious objection, however, are concerned with the extent of one's right to conscientious objection rather than the question of whether a right to conscientious objection exists. One recent example from the United States is that of a nurse working at Vermont medical clinic who in early 2018 was made to participate in the provision of an abortion. The nurse, who is Catholic and who worked at the University of Vermont Medical Center, or UVMMC, had made it clear to her employer that she did not want to participate in abortion procedures for reasons of conscience. According to a complaint filed in May 2018 and a subsequent investigation, her wishes were not honoured. After being told that she would be treating a patient who had experienced a miscarriage, she discovered that she had actually been scheduled to help with an elective abortion. Indeed, a recently created UVMMC policy stated that hospital management can punish staffers who refuse to participate in abortions *when the hospital is short-staffed*. The nurse's supervisor allegedly would not allow her to step out of the procedure. Fearing retaliation, or that she would lose her job, the nurse assisted in the abortion.

In August 2019, the U.S. Health and Human Services Office for Civil Rights (OCR) said that UVMMC broke the law in obliging the nurse to assist in an abortion. The OCR ordered the organisation to change its staffing policy on abortion procedures. UVMMC claimed that the centre "has robust, formal protections that strike the appropriate and legal balance between supporting our employees' religious, ethical, and cultural beliefs, and making sure our patients are not denied access to safe and legal abortion" (UVMMC 2019). The OCR, however, had a different view and ruled that UVMMC had no right to oblige the nurse to participate in the provision of an abortion, even when the hospital was short-staffed (OCR 2019). The right to conscientious objection extends to even these circumstances, the OCR stated.[4]

There have been several other high-profile legal cases in recent years dealing with the scope of the right to conscientious objection in healthcare and, in particular, conscientious objection to abortion. Two hospital midwives in the United Kingdom, for example, had to leave their jobs after the UK Supreme Court ruled in 2014 that they were not allowed to opt out of the rostering of staff to wards responsible for the performance of abortions. Mary Doogan and Concepta Wood had worked as National Health Service (NHS) labour ward co-ordinators at the Southern General Hospital in Glasgow, Scotland, for several decades. In the late 2000s, however, the hospital's labour wards began to offer abortions to patients. Doogan and Wood refused to continue rostering staff to these wards, justifying their objection by invoking a legal right not to participate in abortions in any way. As stated earlier, Section 4 of the Abortion Act 1967 (UK) recognises that conscientious objectors have a right not to participate in the provision of abortions. The two midwives lodged a formal complaint with their employer in September 2009, though this complaint was dismissed as falling beyond the ambit of the Abortion Act. After being dismissed from their work, Doogan and Wood appealed to the courts. The case eventually made its way to the UK Supreme Court, where the legal challenge was unanimously rejected. Lady Hale *et al.* found that the midwives did not have a legal right to object to helping with abortions in any way (UK Supreme Court 2014). The midwives had argued that they should be entitled to refuse to delegate, supervise and support staff involved in the procedures or providing care to patients during the process. Yet the court saw this as an illicit extension of the conscientious objection provisions in the Abortion Act.

Limiting the right to conscientious objection

As the aforementioned case illustrates, some jurisdictions recognise a right to conscientious objection, but this right is subject to significant qualification. For example, referral requirements for abortion are a common feature of abortion law in Australian states and territories (Howe and Le Mire 2019). Similarly, a policy directive on conscientious objection and Medical Assistance in Dying (MAiD) issued in 2016 by the College of Physicians and Surgeons in Ontario, Canada, stated that objecting physicians in the province are obliged to refer patients to other willing medical practitioners who can provide euthanasia (Kelsall 2018; Bodley 2018). A group of physicians in Ontario objected to this directive and took legal action against the college, though the courts found that the referral requirement was a proportionate measure given a patient's right to access MAiD (Court of Appeal for Ontario 2019). Abortion law in some jurisdictions also contains an emergency clause for abortion procedures, whereby doctors and nurses are required to participate in the provision of abortion where a woman's life is at risk. For example, Section 4(2) of the Abortion Act 1967 (UK) states that the right to conscientious objection does not extend to situations in "which [it] is necessary to save the life or to prevent grave permanent injury to the physical or mental health of a pregnant woman".

While legislation is often the ultimate arbiter of whether someone's conscientious objection ought to be tolerated, professional associations also play a role in regulating conscientious objection in healthcare. The British Medical Association, for example, supports a "limited right" to conscientious objection. The organisation "believes that doctors should have a right to conscientiously object to participation in abortion, fertility treatment and the withdrawal of life-sustaining treatment, where there is another doctor willing to take over the patient's care" (BMA 2020). Similarly, the Australian Medical Association's (AMA's) position statement on conscientious objection states that "it is acceptable for a doctor to refuse to provide or to participate in certain medical treatments or procedures based on a conscientious objection". The AMA is of the view, however, that "doctors have an ethical obligation to minimise disruption to patient care and must never use a conscientious objection to intentionally impede patients' access to care" (AMA 2019).

Institutional conscientious objection

Importantly, conscience protections are not limited to individuals but extend in some circumstances to institutions. The right of healthcare institutions to conscientiously object is protected in law in many jurisdictions, in addition to being sanctioned by medical associations. U.S. law, for example, recognises the right of healthcare institutions to refuse to participate in the provision of abortions and voluntary sterilisations. The "Church Amendments" – conscience-based statutes enacted federally in 1973 – state that public funding for religious healthcare facilities should not be conditional on the provision of these services (Bertelsen 2013).

Similarly, euthanasia legislation in South Australia recognises the right of "operators of certain healthcare establishments" to "refuse to authorise or permit the carrying out . . . of any part of the voluntary assisted dying process" (Parliament of South Australia 2021).[5]

Some medical associations also officially recognise the right of institutions to refuse to participate in medical procedures that are contrary to the ethos of the organisation. For example, the AMA recognises institutional conscientious objection as a legitimate form of conscientious objection, though it notes that institutions should notify the public of the services that they do not provide. Other medical associations, such as the American Medical Association, have no official position on the issue of institutional conscientious objection (American Medical Association 2021). To the knowledge of this author, the American Medical Association has been completely silent about the non-participation of religiously affiliated healthcare providers in the provision of services such as abortion. The association remains officially opposed to the practice of voluntary euthanasia and in this respect is in agreement with the position of religiously affiliated healthcare institutions on the provision of euthanasia.

4. Academic debate on conscientious objection and the thesis of this book

So-called conscientious protections – legal or regulatory protections for healthcare professionals who on grounds of conscience refuse to provide or participate in the provision of medical services – have been in place in liberal democracies for many decades. Recently, however, conscience protections have come under increased scrutiny. Ethicists and health experts have raised concern that the practice of conscientious objection is having a negative impact on the delivery of effective and timely medical care to consumers.

In 2005, American legal scholar Alto Charo published an article in the *New England Journal of Medicine* titled "The Celestial Fire of Conscience – Refusing to Deliver Medical Care" (Charo 2005). Charo criticised the monopolisation of care by doctors who in some cases will refuse to provide patients with services that are legal and part of the suite of medical options that licensing bodies expect doctors to provide. Two years later, Australian philosopher Julian Savulescu published an article in the *British Medical Journal* titled "Conscientious Objection in Healthcare", which argued that the practice of conscientious objection opened the door to "a Pandora's box of idiosyncratic, bigoted, discriminatory medicine" (Savulescu 2006). Charo's and Savulescu's articles have been part of the stimulus for a plethora of scholarly works over the past 15 years that have dealt with this topic, many (arguably most) from a critical perspective.

It is not easy to summarise the main themes of the conscientious objection literature as so much has been written on the topic in recent years. Chapter 2 of this book will examine the theoretical underpinnings of arguments against conscientious objection in healthcare. Yet if we were to identify a central claim driving the conscientious objection literature, it would appear to be that many ethicists believe that the primary duty of healthcare professionals is to promote patient welfare and that conscientious objection provisions conflict with this right (Savulescu 2006; Savulescu and Schuklenk 2017; Stahl and Emanuel 2017). That is to say, conscientious objection is seen to be in direct conflict with a physician's respect for patient rights and welfare. Defenders of conscientious objection would argue that conscientious objectors show appropriate concern for patient rights and welfare – they just have a different understanding of what rights and welfare amount to. Yet critics appear to reject this contention and argue that there is a fundamental clash of liberties between doctor and patient when it comes to the matter of conscientious objection.

Related to this, critics of conscientious objection argue that a certain degree of professional detachment is necessary in clinic practice, and this involves being willing to set one's personal beliefs to one side where they conflict with the considered wishes of patients. As such, restrictions on conscientious objection are seen as a necessary and appropriate measure to ensure that patient preferences are respected. From this broad viewpoint, Carolyn McLeod argues in her recent Oxford University Press book *Conscience in Reproductive Healthcare: Prioritising Patient Interests* that healthcare professionals must prioritise patients' preferences over their own ethical or religious beliefs. McLeod argues that healthcare professionals, who are charged with gatekeeping access to services such as abortions, are fiduciaries for their patients and for the public they are licensed to serve. As such, they have a duty of loyalty to these beneficiaries and must give primacy to their interests in gaining access to care (McLeod 2020).[6]

We have also mentioned the issue that many critics of conscientious objection misunderstand or downplay the moral significance of conscience. At the very least, several theorists question the depth with which conscientious objectors hold the beliefs that motivate their objections. Savulescu and Schunklenk, for example, suggest that the conscientious objectors do not think that abortion and euthanasia are wrong in the same way that torture or genocide are wrong. With respect to any objectionable procedure, they write:

> If its rightness or wrongness is of a type or degree that it is a matter of personal preference (ethical relativism), it should not have an impact on patient care.

(2017, 168)

This raises the question of the *costliness* of violating conscience, a topic we will return to later in this book. If Savulescu and Schuklenk are right, then it does not seem unduly costly to violate conscience. What we are dealing with is a matter of superficial preference rather than a matter of fundamental beliefs. As such, we should not be as concerned about the "right to conscientious objection" as we might otherwise be.

Critics may recognise that conscience is important and deserving of respect while still maintaining that physicians ought not to exercise their conscience by the bedside or impose controversial moral views on patients. Many theorists argue that doctors ought to cultivate their consciences through reading widely and educating themselves about the social problems afflicting society and which they might play a role in addressing (Macnaughton 2000; Horton 2019). The issue of racism, for example, has received significant attention in recent bioethics literature, and theorists believe that doctors have a pivotal role to play in addressing systemic racism in the medical system (Peek 2021; Vela, Chin and Peek 2021). Many believe, however, that doctors ought not to impose their personal views on patients when providing care. Doctor-patient interactions ought to be animated by a spirit of liberal neutrality whereby a doctor seeks to promote patient preferences rather than supplanting a patient's preference with their own (Schuklenk and Smalling 2017).

I will argue, however, that one cannot bracket off one's deeply held convictions from one's manner of practising medicine because the exercise of conscience is intrinsic to medical practice. The moral harm that an agent experiences when she seriously contravenes her conscience, furthermore, is much graver than Savulescu and Schuklenk would allow. Indeed, the critique of conscientious objection in recent literature is based on a very thin and under-theorised conception of conscience. In this book, I will challenge the foundational assumptions of recent criticisms of conscientious objection. I will offer a series of objections to the model of medicine that the critique is based on, in addition to criticising the trivialisation of conscience implicit in the work of scholars like Savulescu and Schuklenk.

Conscience is a fundamental feature of human moral psychology, and it is difficult to overestimate its importance. Indeed, I will argue that conscience is a monitor of those commitments that constitute the very horizons of intelligible action for a moral agent. Conscience monitors the extent to which one is acting in accord with a coherent self-conception anchored in a particular understanding of morality and moral duty. That is to say, conscience monitors the extent to which one is living a morally coherent life. Restrictions on the exercise of conscience, however, prevent agents from living in accord with their own convictions and considered understanding of morality. Indeed, we might say that they "fracture the self" and lead to a life in which there is no unifying moral master-narrative. Such a life is one in which one lacks genuine convictions that inform action across personal, social and professional contexts. Such a life, furthermore, is one in which an individual lacks a capacity for moral agency. Moral agency presupposes acting based on a coherent set of principles that one has reflectively endorsed (Frankfurt 1971). But how can one act wholeheartedly if one lacks a coherent set of convictions that transcend the fractured domains of one's life?

In a professional context, conscience is integrally linked to the cultivation of virtue and character, which in turn are essential features of good medical practice. I argue that physicians should have a broad right to exercise their professional discretion and to deliberate based on conscience as to how they ought to act because to do so is not only integral to medical practice but integral to one's humanity. Without space to exercise their agency, physicians will never acquire the character and virtue that are required for the realisation of the goods constitutive of the medical profession. Indeed, the discretionary space of a physician is the moral domain in which a physician's identity is constituted, and where medical ethics goes from being a mere exercise in compliance to constituting the very fabric of one's character. Insofar as we want clinicians to have a deep commitment to fulfilling their professional role and to conscientiously carry out their professional duties, we should protect a physician's discretionary space and his or her right to conscientious objection.

Professional discretion is necessary for doctors to be able to cultivate virtues like care and conscientiousness that we take to be central to the medical profession. A basic assumption motivating my argument is the Aristotelian dictum that virtue cannot just be taught but must also be acquired through activity. Virtues are habits and so become part of the psychology and identity of agents through free and repeated action (cf. Aristotle's *Ethics* 1103a20–1). Physicians must have the opportunity to exercise professional virtue if they are to attain excellence in the fulfilment of their professional role. If physicians cannot act freely, then they cannot be expected to acquire the virtues constitutive of excellence in medical practice.

It is not my intention to argue that the promptings of conscience ought to supplant other sources of normativity in medicine (including the advice of one's peers, professional guidelines, the law and, above all, a patient's needs). I will, however, argue that a practitioner's discretionary judgement should be able to *complement* these sources of normativity. Society has an interest in allowing doctors to preserve their own agential vantage point from which they can independently critique the norms of professional work and social life. That is to say, we have an interest in preserving a doctor's right to call out morally contentious practices that have become accepted features of the profession, at the very least by allowing doctors to opt out of participation in controversial medical procedures.

Lastly, I will argue that the same principles according to which we protect individual conscience ought to be extended to institutional conscience.[7] While I do not believe that institutions have a conscience, there is a sense in which institutional values perform a similar function to the deep commitments that conscience gives voice to in the moral psychology of an agent. If we fail to respect an institution's mission and values – or, more to the point, if we fail to allow an institution to operate in accord with mission and values – then we expose that institution to a kind of moral harm that is analogous to the moral harm experienced by an agent who is coerced into violating their conscience.

5. Some points of clarification

The moral and psychological harm of suppressing conscience

It is important from the outset to distinguish the argument of this book from other arguments in favour of conscience rights that have been made in the public square. Someone might argue that we should never force someone to do something that they know to be wrong. Point 1782 of the *Catechism of the Catholic Church*, for example, states that "man . . . must not be forced to act contrary to his conscience [nor] must he be prevented from acting in accord with his conscience, especially in religious matters". The thought is that conscience is a judgement of reason by which the human person recognises the moral quality of a concrete act and that we ought never to force someone to do something that they know to be immoral. A human being must always obey (and be allowed to obey) the judgements of conscience.

I think it is certainly important that people are not forced to do what they know to be wrong. Yet restrictions on conscience can also fundamentally alter a person's orientation towards morality as such. Restrictions on conscience restrict an agent's ability to act freely in accord with their moral judgements and in doing so may damage an agent's psychological orientation towards acting morally. "Morality" may come to be seen as something imposed from outside and that must be complied with rather than being something that has its origins in empathic concern and one's own moral convictions (sifted through the filter of personal moral reflection and experience or guidance from others). A compliance-based approach to morality runs the risk of effectively turning agents into psychopaths, for indeed psychopaths are precisely called so because they are indifferent towards morality and/or incapable of moral reflection (Vujosevic 2015). Rather, psychopaths only abide by the precepts of morality if they know that they will be punished. This is the primary concern that motivates the argument of this book. We should seek to foster in agents a personal engagement with morality such that they act based on moral principles that they have internalised and that constitute part of their character. Restrictions on the exercise of conscience, however, stultify this process and lead instead to a situation in which moral norms are viewed as an external imposition on one's life that only ought to be obeyed on pain of retribution.

Conscience, relativism and expressive individualism

I should make clear that I am not focusing on conscience to the exclusion of the existence of objective morality. Nor am I neutral on questions pertaining to the morality of abortion or euthanasia or any other medical practice. I am, however, pessimistic about the likelihood that first-order moral debate about the morality of particular procedures will conclude anytime soon. For example, one cannot expect that moral dialogue will lead to a rapid resolution of debate about the moral status of abortion in the near future. I think instead there needs to be a dialogue on meta-ethical questions relevant to the conscientious objection debate. Relevant questions would include the following: "What is the nature of conscience?"; "what are the criteria according to which conscientious objection is deemed morally acceptable?"; and "when is one objecting conscientiously and not merely objecting due to discomfort?". The benefit of focusing on a discussion of conscience is that it holds the promise of progressing this debate beyond first-order discussions of the morality of procedures like abortion or euthanasia.

Is my central thesis a version of what Carter Snead, Carl Trueman and others have labelled *expressive individualism* (Snead 2020; Trueman 2020)? Expressive individualism, in its purest form, asserts that "the individual, atomised self is the fundamental unit of human reality. This self is not defined by its attachments or network of relations, but rather by its capacity to choose a future pathway that is revealed by the investigation of its own inner depths of sentiment. On this view, no object of choice – whether property, a particular vocation, or even the creation of a family – is definitive and constitutive of the self." The self of expressive individualism is, to borrow a phrase from Michael Sandel, an "unencumbered self" (Sandel 1984). Because this self is defined by introspection and acts of self-definition, it is associated fundamentally with its will and not its body. Therefore, expressive individualism is inevitably dualistic and privileges the mind while subordinating the body in defining the person.

I would distinguish the views advanced in this book, however, from expressive individualism. The account of conscience advanced in this book focuses on what I take to be one element of the self – what we might call the existential self or the self that we fashion through our deliberate and sustained life choices – and seeks to explore the implications of this process of self-realisation for the acquisition of virtue and the cultivation of character. I do not mean to deny that the embodied nature of human beings is also integral to a holistic account of the self.[8] I will, however, bracket off reference to the bodily dimensions of the human person in offering my account of conscience.

Indeed, bracketing off of what might otherwise be a controversial claim about human moral psychology provides my argument with broader appeal than it might otherwise have. It is my claim that even those critics who reject a more robust human anthropology (those who reject an embodied account of human personhood and who instead adopt a view analogous to expressive individualism) ought still to accept the basic argument of this book, namely that we ought to respect an agent's fundamental life commitments. One might argue, taking into account movements like MeToo and Black Lives Matter, that we live in an age where standpoint epistemology is in the ascendency. By standpoint epistemology, I have in mind an epistemology that is focused on an individual's personal knowledge and perspectives and the authority (to the exclusion of bias) that comes with first-person testimony. Standpoint epistemologists, furthermore, argue that we ought to show deference for the interests of people in minority categories and ought not to exert power over their experience by attempting to redescribe their experience in terms that might be implicitly oppressive. If indeed standpoint epistemology is in the ascendency, it is quite peculiar that there is so much suspicion attached to motivations of healthcare professionals who make an appeal to conscience in their professional work. At the very least, the standpoint of healthcare professionals ought to be taken seriously and given appropriate weight in debates about professional ethics. Healthcare workers are vulnerable to becoming the unwitting victims of epistemic injustice.

There are, indeed, serious philosophical objections that one might raise about expressive individualism. Snead (2020), for example, suggests that expressive individualism reifies the human will as a means of self-definition instead of focusing on the role that human embodiment plays in providing one with an enduring identity and moral outlook. One's identity risks becoming a mere sentiment or subjective feature of one's self rather than being anchored in the physicality of one's body and one's relationships of dependence and vulnerability vis-à-vis other human beings. This speculation about the shortcomings of expressive individualism, however, goes beyond the scope of the topic at hand.

The scope of my argument

Finally, it is appropriate to discuss the scope of the argument at the centre of this book. Specifically, it is necessary to outline who the argument applies to: physicians alone or healthcare professionals generally. This book will, for the most part, focus on medical professionals. Indeed, Chapter 4 advances a particular account of the nature of medical practice with a view to defending broad conscience protections for physicians. Yet it is not the case that I believe that the exercise of conscience should be permitted in the medical professional alone. Rather, I focus specifically on physicians as I believe that medicine is a paradigm for what we might call "the helping and healing professions" (Pellegrino 2001). That is to say, medicine is of such a nature that many of the ethical claims that we make of it can be readily applied to other healthcare disciplines like nursing, pharmacy and allied health specialties. I will not go as far as to claim that this book demonstrates that all healthcare professionals ought also to be given the right to conscientious objection. But I do not think it would be particularly difficult to extend the arguments advanced in this book to all healthcare professionals. Indeed, it may even be that the case for conscience rights for non-physicians is stronger as they do not fall within the ambit of many of the objections raised by critics of conscientious objection.

It is also useful to clarify what kinds of conscientious objections I will be dealing with in this book. This book will focus on Nature of Medicine Conscientious Objections (NoMCOs) (Kim and Ferguson 2021) – disagreements about how we should think about the goods of medicine in particular situations and how these goods would be best realised – rather than objections based on articles of religion or ethical beliefs that are not concerned with the goods of medicine. I will, for example, be dealing with conscientious objections based on the claim that abortion is bad medicine; I will not, however, be dealing with conscientious objections based on religious tenets such as the religious objection that some Muslim medical doctors have to perform intimate examinations on patients of the opposite sex. I believe that the NoMCO distinction – defended by Kim and Ferguson (2021) – is robust enough to justify this approach. I am not saying that conscientious objections of other kinds should or should not be permitted. I simply set them to one side for the purposes of this book.

6. Precis

It is appropriate to conclude this chapter with a brief summary of the content of the subsequent chapters of this book. In Chapter 2, I explore the theoretical underpinnings of arguments against conscientious objection in healthcare. I focus in particular on the assumptions that critics of conscientious objection make about the nature of medical practice, and I consider the implications of these assumptions for our understanding of medical decision-making and the role of individual practitioner discretion. I discuss the reasons why critics of conscientious objection believe that conscience is morally irrelevant to decision-making in medical practice. This chapter concludes by outlining the case for revising our understanding of the role of conscience in human moral psychology. I contend that conscience is an ethically integral part of the moral psychology of medical practitioners.

The following two chapters are complementary: one discusses why conscience matters in the lives of moral agents, while the other offers a more specific account of the relevance of professional discretionary in medicine to the cultivation of virtue and character. Chapter 3 offers an account of the role of conscience in moral life. I argue that conscience at the most basic level is concerned with a commitment to moral integrity and that restrictions on freedom of conscience prevent agents from living a moral life. I begin by discussing the role of conscience in human moral psychology. I argue that conscience is a principle of moral awareness in rational agents and that it yields an awareness of the personal nature of moral obligation. I discuss the widely endorsed view that conscience monitors the coherence between an agent's self-identifying beliefs and intentions and their practical actions. I then consider how human beings are harmed when they are forced to violate their conscience. Restrictions on the exercise of conscience, I contend, prevent agents from living in accord with their own considered understanding of the requirements of morality. They also undermine certain features of moral rationality that are a prerequisite of agency.

Chapter 4 situates the discussion of conscience within the context of medical practice and makes the case for the accommodation of conscientious objection in medicine. I present an alternative account of medical practice to what Curlin and Tollefsen (2021) call the "provider of services" model of medicine (PSM). In contrast to PSM, I argue that medicine is a goal-directed practice that has as its object the goods of health and healing. I argue that cultivation of character and virtue is essential to realising these goods of medicine and that part of this process involves giving physicians' broad discretion to act in accord with their own considered understanding of good medical practice. Conscience protections are one way of ensuring that a physician's discretionary space is respected.

Chapter 5 considers how we ought to go about accommodating conscientious objectors in medical practice. I discuss existing proposals in the literature for the regulation of conscientious objection, including the idea of a blanket ban on conscientious objection, as well as the contention that we ought to introduce conscience tribunals and referral requirements for conscientious objectors. After critically evaluating these proposals, I discuss a series of alternative proposals, including legislative solutions, a public register, quotas, and doctor-patient matching, that have been put forward as a means to accommodate conscientious objectors at the level of both healthcare administration and clinical practice.

Building on the framework outlined in early chapters, Chapter 6 considers whether institutions have a conscience and whether this matters for the permissibility of conscientious objection. The chapter focuses, in particular, on the costliness of violating deeply held beliefs and considers what relevance this notion might have for our understanding of the ethics of institutional conscientious objection. I offer a brief, metaphysical account of the nature of institutions. I then discuss whether institutions have a conscience. I argue that institutions lack consciousness, and are also not subject to the emotional sanction of conscience, and so cannot be said to have a conscience. Following this, I consider whether the question of conscience matters to the permissibility of institutional conscientious objection. I argue that there are independent reasons for respecting the autonomy and core beliefs of institutions. Institutional liberty is important for the protection of individual conscience. That is to say, institutional liberty is important if we are to respect an individual agent's right to conscientious objection. I also argue that institutional integrity is important for the good of both institutions in themselves and society at large.

Chapter 7 offers some brief concluding remarks on the content discussed in the book and identifies several practical conclusions that policymakers might take from the discussion. I also identify a series of areas of further research that ethicists might consider exploring in future. These relate to both conscience in general and its role in professional life in particular.

Notes

1 See Michael Cook. "An Irish doctor fails in an attempt to be a conscientious objector to Covid-19 policies". *BioEdge* 15 May 2021.
2 Some issues of moral complicity (specifically the issue of complicity and medical referrals) will be discussed in Chapter 5 of this manuscript.
3 With this ruling in view, it is interesting to note that the Council of Europe has recognised a right to conscientious objection for both individuals and institutions. The council passed a resolution in 2010 stating that "no person, hospital or institution shall be coerced, held liable or discriminated against in any manner because of a refusal to perform, accommodate, assist or submit to an abortion" (Parliamentary Council of Europe 2010).
4 Astoundingly, officials appointed to the OCR by the Biden administration quietly reversed this decision and dismissed the case before any corrective action or settlement had taken place (Severino 2021). That is to say, the OCR rescinded its ruling that UVMMC had violated the nurse's right to conscientious objection.
5 "Voluntary assisted dying" is the preferred term for euthanasia in Australian legislation.
6 In the context of this argument, it is worth considering that objecting physicians typically consider a contested procedure to be immoral because it is harmful and, therefore, not in a patient's best interests. Indeed, the law requires physicians to assess the merits of treatment independently and in good faith, using their own judgement, without becoming a "puppet" by taking direction from anyone else, including the patient and state medical regulators. If they thus conclude that doing X is not in a patient's best interest, the law requires them to refuse. See Canadian Aero Service Ltd. v. O'Malley, [1974] SCR 592, 1973 CanLII 23 (SCC) at 606; McInerney v MacDonald, [1992] 2 SCR 138, 1992 CanLII 57 (SCC) at 139, 149, 152; United Kingdom, Law Commission, Report No. 350 Fiduciary Duties of Investment Intermediaries (Williams Lea Group for HM Stationery Office, 2014), Law Commission [UKLCR350] at para 3.53, note 107, citing Selby v Bowie (1863) 8 LT 372, Re Brockbank [1948] Ch 206.
7 For a definition of the term "institution", see Chapter 7.

8 In other words, this book focuses on one's personal identity as a thinking and acting subject rather than one's identity as a rational animal (but I do not deny the embodied aspect of the human person). For a helpful and related discussion of the different accounts of personal identity found in the work of Thomas Aquinas, see John Finnis. "'The thing I am': Personal identity in Aquinas and Shakespeare". *Social Philosophy and Policy* 22(2) (2005): 250–282.

References

American Medical Association. *Code of Medical Ethics*. Chicago: American Medical Association, 2021.

Australian Medical Association. *AMA Position Statement on Conscientious Objection*. Sydney: Australian Medical Association, 2019.

Barczak, Eleanor. "Ethical implications of the conscience clause on access to postpartum tubal ligations". *Hastings Law Journal* 70;6 (2019): 1613–1638.

Bertelsen, S. "Conscientious objection of health care providers: Lessons from the experience of the United States". *Notre Dame Journal of International and Comparative Law* 10;1 (2013): 122–148.

Bodley, Steven. "The College of Physicians and Surgeons of Ontario on MAiD referrals". *Canadian Medical Association Journal* 190;23 (2018): E724.

Boulware, David, Pullen, Matthew, Bangdiwala, Ananta *et al.* "A randomized trial of hydroxychloroquine as postexposure prophylaxis for covid-19". *New England Journal of Medicine* 383 (2020): 517–525.

British Medical Association. *Expressing your Personal Beliefs as a Doctor*. London: British Medical Association, 2020. Available from www.bma.org.uk/advice-and-support/ethics/personal-ethics/expressing-your-personal-beliefs-as-a-doctor.

Butler, Joseph. *Fifteen Sermons Preached at the Rolls Chapel*. London: Botham, 1950 [1726].

Callahan, Daniel. "Bioethics and the culture wars". *Cambridge Quarterly of Healthcare Ethics* 14;4 (2005): 424–431.

Catholic Church. *Catechism of the Catholic Church*. Vatican City: Libreria Editrice Vaticana, 1992.

Charo, Alta. "The celestial fire of conscience: Refusing to deliver medical care". *New England Journal of Medicine* 352 (2005): 2471–2473.

Court of Appeal of Ontario. Christian Medical and Dental Society of Canada v. College of Physicians and Surgeons of Ontario. 2019 *ONCA* 393.

Curlin, Farr, and Tollefsen, Christopher. *The Way of Medicine: Ethics and the Healing Profession*. South Bend: University of Notre Dame Press, 2021.

Durland, Spenser. "The case against institutional conscientious objection". *Notre Dame Law Review* 86;4 (2011): 1655–1686.

Finnis, John. "'The thing I am': Personal identity in Aquinas and Shakespeare". *Social Philosophy and Policy* 22;2 (2005): 250–282.

Frankfurt, Harry. "Freedom of the will and the concept of a person". *Journal of Philosophy* 68 (1971): 5–20.

Fuss, Peter. "Conscience". *Ethics* 74;2 (1964): 111–120.

Hoffmann, Tobias. "Conscience and synderesis". In Brian Davies (ed.). *The Oxford Handbook of Aquinas*. London: Oxford University Press, 2012: 255–262.

Horton, Mary E. Kollmer. "The orphan child: Humanities in modern medical education". *Philosophy, Ethics, and Humanities in Medicine* 14 (2019): 1.

Howe, Joanna, and Le Mire, Suzanne. "Medical referral for abortion and freedom of conscience in Australian Law". *Journal of Law and Religion* 34;1 (2019): 85–112.

Kelsall, Diane. "Physicians are not solely responsible for ensuring access to medical assistance in dying". *Canadian Medical Association Journal* 190;7 (2018): E181.

Keogh, Louise, Gillam, Lynn, Bismark, Marie, *et al.* "Conscientious objection to abortion, the law and its implementation in Victoria, Australia: Perspectives of abortion service providers". *BMC Medical Ethics* 20;11 (2019): 1–10.

Kheriaty, Aaron. "Legal case". (2021). Available from www.aaronkheriaty.com/work.

Kim, Eric, and Ferguson, Kyle. "Conscientious objection, the nature of medicine, and the need for reformability". *Bioethics* first published 31st August 2021. doi: 10.1111/bioe.12943.

King, Louise. "Sex selection for non-medical reasons". *AMA Journal of Ethics* 9;6 (2007): 418–422.

Kirby, J. "Should institutional conscientious objection to assisted dying be accommodated?". *Canadian Journal of Bioethics* 4;1 (2021): 15–20.

Macnaughton, Jane. "The humanities in medical education: Content, outcomes and structures". *British Medical Journal* 26 (2000): 23–30.

McLeod, Carolyn. *Conscience in Reproductive Healthcare: Prioritising Patient Interests.* New York: Oxford University Press, 2020.

Munthe, Christian. "Conscientious refusal in healthcare: The Swedish solution". *Journal of Medical Ethics* 43;4 (2017): 257–259.

Nelson, Lawrence. "Provider conscientious refusal of abortion, obstetrical emergencies, and criminal homicide law". *The American Journal of Bioethics* 18;7 (2018): 43–50.

Office for Civil Rights. "OCR issues notice of violation to the University of Vermont Medical Center after it unlawfully forced a nurse to assist in abortion". Washington, DC: Health and Human Services, 2019. Available from www.hhs.gov/guidance/document/ocr-issues-notice-violation-university-vermont-medical-center-after-it-unlawfully-forced.

Parliament of South Australia. *Voluntary Assisted Dying Act 2021.* Adelaide: Government of South Australia. Available from www.legislation.sa.gov.au/__legislation/lz/c/a/voluntary%20assisted%20dying%20act%202021/current/2021.29.auth.pdf.

Parliamentary Assembly of the Council of Europe. "Resolution 1763: The right to conscientious objection in lawful medical care". Brussels: Council of Europe, 2010.

Peek, Monica. "Black history is America's history". *EClinicalMedicine* 32 (2021): 100755.

Pellegrino, Edmund. "The internal morality of clinical medicine: A paradigm for the ethics of the helping and healing professions". *The Journal of Medicine and Philosophy* 26;6 (2001): 559–579.

Rousseau, Jean Jacques. *Emile: Or On Education.* Barbara Foxley (trans.). London & Toronto: J.M. Dent and Sons, 1921 [1762].

Sandel, Michael. "The procedural republic and the unencumbered self". *Political Theory* 12;1 (1984): 81–96.

Savulescu, Julian. "Conscientious objection in medicine". *British Medical Journal* 332 (2006): 294.

Savulescu, Julian, and Schuklenk, Udo. "Doctors have no right to refuse medical assistance in dying, abortion or contraception". *Bioethics* 31;3 (2017): 162–170.

Schuklenk, Udo. "Conscientious objection in medicine: Accommodation versus professionalism and the common good". *British Medical Bulletin* 126;1 (2018): 47–56.

Schuklenk, Udo, and Smalling, Ricardo. "Why medical professionals have no moral claim to conscientious objection accommodation in liberal democracies". *Journal of Medical Ethics* 43 (2017): 234–240.

Severino, Roger. "Becerra and Biden betray medical professionals being forced to assist in abortions". *The National Review* 3rd August 2021. Available from www.nationalreview.com/corner/becerra-and-biden-betray-medical-professionals-being-forced-to-assist-in-abortions/.

Snead, Carter. *What It Means to Be Human: The Case for the Body in Public Bioethics.* Cambridge: Harvard University Press, 2020.

Stahl, Ronit, and Emanuel, Ezekiel. "Physicians, not conscripts – conscientious objection in healthcare". *New England Journal of Medicine* 376 (2017): 1380–1385.

Strickland, Sophie. "Conscientious objection in medical students: A questionnaire survey". *Journal of Medical Ethics* 38 (2012): 22–25.

Sulmasy, Daniel. "What is conscience and why is respect for it so important". *Theoretical Medicine and Bioethics* 29 (2008): 135–149.

Trueman, Carl. *The Rise and Triumph of the Modern Self: Cultural Amnesia, Expressive Individualism and the Road to the Sexual Revolution.* Wheaton: Crossway, 2020.

UK Supreme Court. Greater Glasgow Health Board (Appellant) v Doogan and another (Respondents) (Scotland). 2014 *UKSC* 68.

University of Vermont Medical Centre. "UVM Medical Center's response to HHS' Office of Civil Rights announcement". Burlington: UVM Medical Centre, 2019. Available from https://twitter.com/UVMMedCenter/status/1166799484359237632.

Vela, Monica, Chin, Marshall, and Peek, Monica. "Keeping our promise – supporting trainees from groups that are underrepresented in medicine". *New England Journal of Medicine* 385;6 (2021): 487–489.

Victorian Government. *Voluntary Assisted Dying Act 2017.* Melbourne, Victorian Government, 2017. Available from www.health.vic.gov.au/patient-care/voluntary-assisted-dying.

Vujosevic, Marijana. "Conscience as the rational deficit of psychopaths". *Philosophical Psychology* 28;8 (2015): 1219–1240.

White, Ben, Wilmott, Lindy, Downie, Jocelyn *et al.* "Legislative options to address institutional objections to voluntary assisted dying in Australia". *UNSW Law Journal Forum* 3 (2021): 1–19.

Wolfe, Robert M., and Sharpe, Lisa K. "Antivaccinationists past and present". *British Medical Journal* 325 (2002): 430.

2 Conscience under fire

A critical analysis of the case against conscientious objection in medicine

Introduction

This chapter explores the theoretical underpinnings of arguments against conscientious objection in healthcare. I focus in particular on the professional duties of healthcare professionals. Section 1 outlines a series of assumptions that critics of conscientious objection make about the nature of medical practice and the duties of doctors. Critics of conscientious objection variously describe doctors as "service providers", "public servants" and "physicians, not conscripts". They also describe doctors as "fiduciaries" who ought to make the values of patients their own, rather than imposing their own personal values on patients (McLeod 2020). Section 2 considers how these assumptions motivate criticism of conscientious objection. If indeed doctors are service providers who ought to pay moral deference to professional standards and patient values, then it seems that conscientious objection ought to be heavily restricted if allowed at all. Section 3, however, outlines the case for revising our understanding of the role of conscience in human moral psychology and medical practice. I contend that conscience is integral to moral life and plays a central role in medical decision-making. This discussion sets the scene for the following two chapters which provide a detailed account of the role of conscience in moral life and in medical practice.

This chapter is not a detailed summary of different arguments against conscientious objection. There are two reasons why I have chosen not to summarise recent literature on conscientious objection. First, focusing on assumptions underpinning arguments against conscientious objection helps us to get at the core of the problem with conscientious objection rather than becoming preoccupied with the minutiae of arguments. Second, it would be difficult to offer an adequate summary of the academic literature considering how much the literature has burgeoned in recent years. For these reasons, I will focus on the theoretical underpinnings of arguments against conscientious objection.

1. Contemporary assumptions about medical practice

This section analyses a series of assumptions that critics of conscientious objection make about the nature of medical practice and the role of medical practitioners.

DOI: 10.4324/9781003247623-2

Critics of conscientious objection variously describe doctors as "service providers", "public servants" and "physicians, not conscripts". McLeod (2020) describes doctors as fiduciaries who ought to advocate for patient values in the domain of medical practice. To be clear, my intention in this section is to offer a clear articulation of the assumptions underpinning arguments against conscientious objection; I do *not* endorse these assumptions. I will, however, attempt to give the strongest possible formulation of these claims so as to avoid any accusation that I have "strawmanned" my interlocutors or misrepresented arguments in the literature.

Doctors as service providers and public servants

It is appropriate to begin our discussion with an overview of the model of medicine that underpins at least some mainstream critiques of conscientious objection in medicine. We might usefully call this the provider of services model of medicine (PSM) (Tollefsen and Curlin 2019), while noting that this title may fail to capture some of the complexities of arguments in the literature. PSM situates medical practice within the context of a liberal democracy and a market economy. Citizens have a presumptive right to healthcare access, including a right to reproductive healthcare, a right to have one's sexual identity recognised and therapeutically affirmed, a right to die and so on. This right to healthcare is akin to other basic rights that a citizen has, such as a right to education, a right to legal representation and a right to private property. PSM places significant weight on the idea of *service provision*. We might think of medicine as a service akin to other services provided in society such as the provision of legal services or the provision of cleaning services. In the case of medicine, doctors provide *healthcare*. Healthcare should be understood in a broad sense and should include not only therapeutic interventions but also any intervention that may be thought to be conducive to patient well-being. According to PSM, the function of medicine in a liberal democracy is to provide healthcare services that are safe and legal to the general public. The medical profession exists to meet the health needs of society. This is the basis of the structure that it has, the government support that it receives and the licensing processes that underpin it (Sulmasy 2017; Cholbi 2018). Indeed, the success or failure of medicine as a profession should be measured by the extent to which it fulfils this role.

This is not to deny that medicine is a profession. Medicine *is* a profession, at least insofar as it involves an ordered body of technical knowledge put to the service of the public interest. Doctors train for many years to gain an adequate grasp of the medical art and to provide care that is safe and efficacious. They are then licensed and initiated into the profession. Upon entering medicine, doctors *profess* to act in the patient's best interest and to be responsible and diligent as medical practitioners. They commit to setting their own personal interests aside and to be an advocate for the interests of their patients, or so it might be argued. This detachment and commitment to patients are the essence of medical professionalism (Stahl and Emanuel 2017, 1384).[1]

Medicine is also sometimes described as an *essential service*. Indeed, medicine is a vital service for society, in contrast to other consumer services like pool cleaning or tattoo artistry. The average citizen will not be seriously affected if he or she is unable to contract a pool cleaner or receive a tattoo. Many people will, however, be seriously affected if they are unable to access adequate medical care. The medical profession exists to meet a basic need of society, and the well-being of a population suffers if medical practitioners fail to fulfil their role.

Yet it is precisely because medicine is an essential service that its success should be measured in terms of the comprehensiveness and quality of healthcare coverage in the community. That is, the success of medicine should be determined by the extent to which it provides a comprehensive suite of medical interventions to patients and provides these services in a timely and convenient fashion. Medical professionals have monopoly control over medical care. If they fail to fulfil their role, they are undermining medicine's raison d'être and failing to act in the public interest.

Doctors are, in many if not most cases, performing the role of public servants, or so it is argued. As Michael Cholbi (2018) observes, "the professions in which conscientious refusal is invoked nearly always operate as public cartels. They enjoy various economic benefits, including protection from competition, that are made possible by governments exercising their powers of coercion, regulation and taxation." This protection is provided because medicine and other healthcare professions provide a vital social service – a service the government has an interest in ensuring that it is provided reliably. Indeed, in many countries healthcare is socialised, such that almost all clinicians are employees of state-run companies or trusts. In the United Kingdom, for example, the vast majority of registered medical practitioners are employed in some capacity by the NHS, with a small number of clinicians in specialities such as oncology, orthopaedics and cosmetic surgery working solely in private practice. Clinicians occupying a public role – such as doctors employed by the NHS – are in many ways similar to public servants working in other branches of government (Savulescu 2006).

If doctors are acting as *employees of the state*, then they ought to deliver healthcare in a manner compatible with the standards and values of the state. Doctors should not attempt to import their own values into healthcare practice. Rather, they should deliver services that are sanctioned by relevant state authorities. A failure to deliver appropriate, state-sanctioned professional services, according to Cholbi (2018), would amount to a form of disrespect of the profession's clients and would be in opposition to liberal ideals of political neutrality. An obstetrician and gynaecologist who refused to provide elective abortions, for example, would be acting in a morally paternalistic way towards their patients and would be undermining an ethos of liberal tolerance in medicine.

This understanding of the role of doctors does not go as far as to suppose that medical practitioners are mere *apparatchiks of the state*. Everyone, critics and proponents of conscientious objection alike, recognises that some amount of professional discretion is required vis-à-vis the advisability of medical treatment in a particular situation, the evidence base supporting a novel intervention and so on.[2]

Professional detachment does not equal professional passivity. It may even be the case that critics of conscientious objection accept that conscience is a crucial part of decision-making in most morally charged contexts. The issue is not with people using their consciences but on working out what to do with physicians whose consciences guide judgements or behaviour that would undermine patient welfare and autonomy (as well as democratically established rules for good medicine).

The ambit of professional discretion does not extend to contentious questions of value in medicine such as whether services such as an abortion, euthanasia or emergency contraceptives ought to be made available to patients. Where these questions of value are concerned, doctors ought to practise in accord with the values of the state and relevant medical authorities as well as the considered preferences of their patients. Any other approach would contravene one's responsibility as a public servant and an advocate for the interests of one's patients.

PSM stands in stark contrast to a more traditional model of medicine and medical care. The former has no implicit orientation towards human goods like health and the relief of suffering (Omelianchuk 2018, 372). Rather, medicine exists to provide a broad range of services, some of which may be concerned with health but many of which have nothing at all to do with health (at least not in a therapeutic sense of the word). In contemporary medical practice, patients routinely request interventions that are not strictly conducive to health and healing. Contraceptives, for example, are typically prescribed with the intent of allowing a patient to avoid unwanted conception. They are not intended to remedy or prevent a particular pathology; they may not even be prescribed for the purpose of protecting a patient against sexually transmitted diseases. As such, they have nothing to do with healing or the prevention of illness. Rather, they are intended to provide sexual autonomy to a patient.[3] Similarly, euthanasia – which is now legal in many jurisdictions around the world – involves the active ending of the life of a patient. This is contrary to traditional medico-ethical maxim that doctors ought above all to refrain from harming a patient. Yet euthanasia is given the labels of *medical assistance in dying* and *voluntary assisted dying*. It is characterised as a medical intervention in jurisdictions where it has been legalised, and several theorists argue that euthanasia is part of basic healthcare. This is another example of why one might be sceptical about a "rigid" account of medicine focused on the goods of health and the relief of suffering.

In summary, the role of a physician, according to PSM, is to provide safe and legal medical services to patients regardless of whether or not these services conflict with the physician's deeply held beliefs. Physicians represent the state, and their primary function is to provide services in a reliable manner and in accord with the values and expectations of the state. Anything less than this would amount to dereliction of duty.

"Physicians, not conscripts"

So far we have considered how doctors might be viewed as representatives of the state who are employed to provide an essential service. Another way in which some scholars conceptualise the responsibilities of medical practitioners is by comparing (and contrasting) their role with that of conscripted soldiers in the military. Stahl and Emanuel suggest that conscientious objection is a concept, the origins of which can be traced back to the practice of conscription in the 19th and 20th centuries (Stahl and Emanuel 2017, 1380).[4] Conscientious objectors were those conscripted soldiers who refused to occupy combat roles in war and were as a result either reassigned to another role, censured by military authorities and/or discharged from duty. Sometimes conscientious objectors were allowed to avoid military service by finding replacements or by paying fines. In the United States, for example, legislatures have historically allowed recognised religious pacifists, such as Quakers, to avoid bearing arms by hiring substitute soldiers or paying substantial fines (Stahl and Emanuel 2017, 1380). In the United Kingdom, the Military Service Act 1916, which introduced conscription for men aged 18 to 41 years, included a conscience clause whereby men could apply to be recognised as conscientious objectors and either serve in a non-combatant role or are exempted from military service altogether (UK Parliament 2021). One need not be religious to be recognised as a conscientious objector under the act. Conscientious objectors, however, sometimes faced harsh penalties such as being denied the right to vote for several years following the First World War.

Are medical professionals in the same situation as conscripted military personnel? Critics of conscientious objection in medicine point out that doctors have voluntarily entered medicine in contrast to soldiers who have been conscripted into the military. One could argue that conscripted soldiers deserve the right to conscientiously object as they may have been co-opted into military service rather than voluntarily agreeing to serve in combat (Cohen 1968). Doctors, in contrast, are engaged in a voluntary professional undertaking, and no one is forcing them to remain in the profession. One cannot marshal the same pro-conscience rhetoric that animated anti-war protests in the 1960s and 1970s and apply this to contemporary debates about the obligations of healthcare professionals, or so it might be argued. Conscientious objectors to the Vietnam War were engaged in a form of protest to what they perceived to be an unjust war. Indeed, conscientious objection ultimately was one of the factors that led to the collapse of the draft system in the United States (Raley 2020). In contrast, there is nothing morally admirable about a medical professional who is refusing to provide essential medical services to patients. Worse, it would be an unmitigated disaster if conscientious objection severely undermined the reliability of the healthcare system. The two situations are very different, then, and we should be wary of surreptitious attempts to justify conscientious objection in medicine on the same grounds as conscientious objection to wartime service.

Indeed, one might argue that there is a contract that doctors tacitly consent to when they enter the profession. They "know what they are getting into". Thus, Schuklenk and Smalling write,

> Anyone joining a profession knows, or should know, that it is ultimately up to society to determine the scope of professional practice.
>
> (2017, 238)

The basic claim here is that licensed doctors agree to provide the full suite of medical services that is considered by society to be part of basic medical care. They undertake to provide healthcare – as determined by patients and the medical profession – in a reliable fashion.

A corollary of this is that doctors should accept the consequences of their actions if they fail to honour patient preferences. If a doctor cannot deliver services reliably, and they lack a valid exculpatory reason, then they should be prepared to leave the profession. As Schuklenk and Smalling (2017, 238) write, "professionals can be expected to take responsibility for the voluntary choices they make". This is the case even when the reason for a doctor not fulfilling their professional role is moral conflict. Someone who enters the medical profession should be prepared to fulfil their duties as a medical practitioner, whether these be professional responsibilities in general or moral responsibilities in particular.

One exception to this rule might be physicians who have been involved in medicine for many decades and who entered medicine at a time when medico-ethical norms were very different. It may be the case, for example, that a physician entered medicine at time when abortion and euthanasia were not commonplace in medical practice and, in any case, physicians were given significant discretionary liberties about how they chose to practise the art of medicine. One could argue that older physicians are to some extent in a similar position to conscripted soldiers, at least insofar as they are part of an institution that has evolved to such an extent that it now is predicated on completely different values to the physician's own values (Savulescu and Schuklenk 2017, 163).

Yet as a general rule, it remains the case that physicians ought to respect the values of the profession even where these values diverge from their own moral code. Presuming that individual physicians have not been the unwitting victims of radical paradigm changes in medicine, then they should seek to practise in accord with the current values that underpin medical practice. Either that, or they should seek an alternative means of employment (Clarke 2017, 220). Practitioners who joined medicine when different expectations were in play can be "grandfathered out" of the profession (Savulescu and Schuklenk 2017, 163).

Many also argue that an attempt to put a doctor's personal preferences first would be tantamount to a violation of patient autonomy. To understand this latter claim, it is apposite to now turn our attention to the fiduciary responsibilities of medical practitioners.

Doctors as fiduciaries

Another conception of the role of a physician in the literature is the *fiduciary model of medical practice*. Some theorists argue that doctors have fiduciary responsibilities towards their patients (Hui 2005; Mehlman 2015; McLeod 2020). A fiduciary is someone who is entrusted with significant discretionary power by another and is given authority over significant practical interests of the other (sometimes known as *the beneficiary*). They are obliged to act in a manner that is reflective of their beneficiary's interests. In the case of medicine, doctors are called on by their patients to pursue the medical good and to identify and carry out interventions that will be conducive to a patient's well-being.

To be clear, there is a significant power differential between doctors and patients as patients are not able to act as doctors themselves. Patients must instead entrust their health interests to a representative or fiduciary who will act on their behalf and pursue such health interests.[5] Thus, McLeod writes:

> Th[e] fiduciary relationship involves a distinctive kind of power: that is, authority to set or promote significant practical interests of another, usually within a certain sphere. This power engenders a certain type of vulnerability: structural vulnerability to the misuse or abuse of discretionary authority over one's significant practical interests.
>
> (p. 123)

Patients invest a huge amount of authority in doctors every time they seek healthcare. With this investment of authority come responsibilities on the part of doctors. Doctors, McLeod argues, must not impose their own preferences on patients but rather must seek to promote the interests of patients regardless of how these interests conflict with their own.[6]

This relationship of trust and vulnerability gives rise to certain obligations for physicians. Physicians cannot just act however they wish regardless of how this impacts on the patient. One should not assume that a fiduciary relationship sanctions what McLeod calls fiduciary paternalism or the exercise of physician discretionary judgement in a manner that ignores the considered preferences of patients. On the contrary, physicians have a moral duty to put the interests of patients first and to seek to realise these interests through the use of their professional expertise.

We might describe this primary commitment of a fiduciary as one of *fidelity*. That is to say, the primary duty of a fiduciary is one of fidelity or loyalty to their beneficiary. This duty requires fiduciaries to devote themselves to serving their beneficiaries' interests within the sphere of the authority that is vested in them (McLeod 2020, 124). Fidelity for physicians is about being faithful to one's patient and promoting their interests. It is about making the patient's preferences one's own, rather than filtering the patient's preferences through one's own moral lens and determining whether their preferences ought to be honoured or not. Such an approach, according to McLeod, would lead us back to fiduciary paternalism and would be a form of false faithfulness.

There are both conceptual and moral reasons as to why pursuing the interests of beneficiaries is important for a fiduciary. Conceptually, for fiduciaries to act on behalf of their beneficiaries, they must pursue the interests of their beneficiaries rather than pursuing their own interests. One acts on someone's behalf only if one acts in that person's interests, which in turn involves acting in accordance with what the person has authorised one to do (Hahn Chaet 2017, 676). But there are also moral reasons one might give for the duty of loyalty. Loyalty is the appropriate moral response of a fiduciary who has been given discretionary authority over a vulnerable third party. Beneficiaries are at serious risk of exploitation by fiduciaries: that is, they are at serious risk of fiduciaries taking unfair advantage of them in their vulnerable state. That is true because of the knowledge gap between them and their fiduciaries and also because of the discretion fiduciaries have. The knowledge gap makes it easy for fiduciaries to convince beneficiaries that a certain course of action advances their interests when objectively speaking it does not. In addition, the discretion fiduciaries have in deciding how to advance their beneficiaries' interests gives them room to convince themselves that they are furthering these interests when instead they are promoting their own interests or those of a third party. This last point helps to explain the concern that some scholars have about exploitation in the fiduciary relationship as well as the rule, common in medicine, that fiduciaries ought to avoid conflicts of interest (Parker *et al*. 2011). In the following section, we will consider how some scholars conceptualise conscientious objection as a conflict of interest (COI).

2. The purported impermissibility of conscientious objection in medicine

In this section, I will consider why a conception of physicians as service providers, willing members of the medical profession and fiduciaries might lead one to conclude that conscientious objection should be heavily restricted if allowed at all. There are two basic elements to the critique of conscientious objection in the literature: First, critics argue that the law and professional standards ought to take precedence over a physician's values; second, doctors should put patient values ahead of their own personal beliefs. I will discuss these two elements in turn.

Law and professional norms take priority over a physician's values

Critics of conscientious objection argue that a physician's practices vis-à-vis controversial procedures such as abortion and euthanasia should be determined by democratically established norms of the profession (Stahl and Emanuel 2017, 1382). Professions associations, for example, ought to be the final arbiters of whether physicians should or should not provide morally contentious services (and under what conditions). Physicians should not bring their own subjective values to bear on whether or not they will provide particular medical services. Rather, they should set their values aside and practise in accord with relevant professional standards (Stahl and Emanuel 2017, 1382).

As we have seen, some theorists argue that physicians are best described as service providers (Savulescu 2006, 294; Stahl and Emanuel 2017, 1383) while others suggest that physicians are public servants (Cholbi 2018). If a physician is a service provider, they ought to provide the service that society expects them to provide. The nature of this service, and the manner in which it should be provided, is best determined by relevant professional associations, lawmakers and relevant government bodies. Indeed, if physicians are employees of the state, that is all the more reason for them to conform to relevant law and professionals standards vis-à-vis practices such as abortion and euthanasia. An analogy might be a county clerk who refuses to certify same-sex marriages. The role of a clerk is to certify contracts such as marriages that have been contracted in accord with the law and in good faith. The clerk should not decide which civil contracts they personally deem to be ethical and worthy of sanction. Rather, they should act in accordance with the laws and regulations of the jurisdiction in which they work. This is what it means for a public servant to fulfil their role (Kim 2016). Public servants, in other words, ought not to seek to conscientiously object to the provision of safe and legal medical procedures. Rather, they should practise in accord with the laws of the state and extant professional ethical guidelines.

In the case of medicine, it could be argued that the contract that physicians enter into includes a commitment to carrying out those tasks that profession deems to be essential. Medicine is not a profession where doctors can "offer partial medical services or partially discharge their obligations to care for their patients" (Savulescu 2006, 294). Rather,

> [i]f a service a doctor is requested to perform is a medical practice, is legal, consistent with distributive justice, requested by the patient or their appointed surrogate, and is plausibly in their interests, the doctor must ensure the patient has access to it.
>
> (Savulescu and Schuklenk 2017, 168)

Anything other than this would be a violation of a doctor's professional duties, or so critics argue. Without appropriate professional standards in place, doctors may practise in a manner that is highly idiosyncratic and that would set a dangerous precedent for dissent in medicine (Schuklenk and Smalling 2017, 234–236). If all doctors were conscientious objectors, it would be difficult to achieve any form of uniformity in medical practice. Rather, practitioners would be endlessly introducing their own subjective values into the provision of medical care and routinely undermining the satisfaction of patient preferences. Thus, Savulescu writes: "the door to 'value-driven medicine' is a door to a Pandora's box of idiosyncratic, bigoted, discriminatory medicine" (Savulescu 2006, 297). In addition, conscientious objection could be said to provide a justification for negligence in medical practice. Derelictions of duty could be passed off as exercises of practitioner' rights. Practitioners could opt out of procedures they simply find distasteful or burdensome by claiming that they have a conscientious objection to such practices.[7]

To be clear, the claim is not that doctors ought to blindly suppress their conscience and mindlessly conform to relevant professional standards. The concern rather is that doctors need to be prepared to deal with the physical and psychological challenges that are inherent in their profession. They cannot absent themselves from their professional role when they find aspects of their work difficult or confronting. As Savulescu and Schuklenk (2017, 164) write:

> Doctors must put patients' interests ahead of their own integrity. They must ensure that legal, beneficial, desired services are provided, if not by them, then by others.

This is in essence what it means to be a conscientious healthcare professional. Conscientious objectors, on the other hand, are arguably failing to fulfil their professional duties when they absent themselves from performing procedures such as abortion or providing a patient with assistance in suicide. They abandon their patients when they need them most rather than accompanying them through the trials of ill health and injury.

Indeed, it could be argued that in medicine we have a problem of dirty hands whereby a doctor is compelled to engage in practices that they deem personally objectionable but that are necessary to bring about a greater good (Walzer 1992; Berlinger 2015). The *problem of dirty hands* is typically concerned with whether political leaders are justified in committing (gravely) immoral actions when this is necessary to realise some important moral or political end, such as the preservation of a community's continued existence or the prevention of imminent societal catastrophe (Walzer 1992, 259). Doctors may not like the realities of medicine where they have to deal with a variety of patients with complex life situations and who bring to the medical encounter their own unique set of values. But in a situation where patients need treatments to improve their own physical and (more to the point) psychological well-being, doctors ought to comply. Ideological and moral purity is the privilege of doctors who refuse to join their patients in the moral quagmires of life. Such an attitude is unbecoming of a conscientious physician.

Finally, it could be argued that conscientious objection amounts to a COI that impedes a doctor's capacity to fulfil his or her professional role. COIs in medicine are typically taken to be financial in nature: it is often assumed that a COI occurs when a healthcare practitioner's financial interest conflicts with patients' interests, public health interests or professional obligations more generally. Yet Giubilini and Savulescu (2020) argue that problematic conflicts of interest may also be non-financial in nature. Specifically, they argue that conscientious objection amounts to a non-financial COI whereby a physician's personal values come into conflict with their professional obligations. "Allowing conscientious objection means precisely allowing certain well identified personal religious or moral views to affect one's professional practice" (2020, 239), the authors argue. This leads to the violation of patients' rights and ought not to be allowed. Rather, the authors argue that "where a doctor's personal values conflict with the accepted professional and ethical standards, they should be disclosed" (2020, 241). "Healthcare professionals", furthermore, "should provide [any] agreed service if it is medically indicated and in line with professional standards" (2020, 241). This is what professional duty requires of physicians with a moral objection to certain procedures.[8]

Doctors should put patient values ahead of their own personal beliefs

As discussed in the previous section, doctors are fiduciaries for their patients. They should seek to promote their patients' values rather than acting based on personal belief. Doctors should recognise the position of vulnerability that their patients are in. The decision by a doctor to refuse a patient's request for safe and legal services is all the more egregious because of the power differential that exists between doctors and patients. Doctors should be aware of this and refrain from letting their own personal values determine what services a patient is given access to.

McLeod (2020) stresses that conscientious objectors are gatekeepers in the healthcare system, and it is only with the consent of doctors that patients can access the medical services that they want and need. McLeod argues that doctors have an obligation arising from their role as fiduciaries to prioritise patient interests and to provide the services that a patient requests. Either that, or they should direct the patient to another clinician who is willing to provide the said service. For McLeod, the relevant virtue is one of fidelity to one's patients, whereby a doctor seeks to discharge their responsibility as a fiduciary by faithfully seeking to advance the "significant practical interests" of their patient (2020, 123). Fidelity means that physicians ought to "put their patients' health interests first, ahead of their own interests" (2020, 126). It is precisely because doctors are in a fiduciary relationship with their patients that they have a special duty to promote their patients' interests. The idea of fiduciary paternalism – whereby a doctor feels the obligation to guide their patients' judgements – is, according to McLeod, a deeply misguided interpretation of what it means to be a dutiful fiduciary.

One could argue for a middle ground whereby the doctor-patient relationship is conceptualised as an *exchange of values*, in which both the doctor's values and the patient's values are brought to bear on a particular situation. Pellegrino, for example, described the doctor – patient encounter as a meeting of "life-worlds" in which the vulnerable patient, sick or injured, seeks help from the doctor, who professes to be a healer (Pellegrino 2004). In this encounter, the doctor commits to act for the good of the patient and seeks, where possible, to restore the patient to health.

Yet, in the end, a patient's values ought to win out whenever there is a conflict between the will of a patient and the values of a doctor. Conscientious objection involves medical practitioners usurping patient rights and going proxy for the better judgement of patients. Conscientious objectors impede the provision of services to which patients are entitled, all in the name of highly dubious and subjective values that ultimately have no place in medicine. At best, conscientious objectors are deeply confused about their own professional duties and fail to recognise the extent to which a principle of patient autonomy overrides other relevant medical considerations. At worst, they are engaged in a form of "cultural conquest" which severely limits patient access to medical services and does deep harm to them in the process (Charo 2005, 2743). In the end, when we are dealing with contentious medical procedures (for example, abortion and euthanasia) doctors should be prepared to defer to the values of their patients.

We should bear in mind that patient autonomy has steadily come to replace physician paternalism as the overriding principle for decision-making in contemporary medicine. As Kilbride and Joffe observe, "the rejection of medical paternalism in favor of respect for patient autonomy transformed the patient-physician relationship" (2018, 1973–1974). Rather than enforcing their own will on patients, doctors now defer to patient preferences and consent when determining what interventions ought to be provided. It stands to reason, then, that doctors ought to defer to patients when they request controversial medical procedures which may conflict with one's own personal values. Indeed, one could argue that there is even more reason for doctors to defer to patient wishes when we are dealing with more value-laden decisions in medicine. The case for refusing to provide care for a patient is weaker when we are talking about abortion or euthanasia, which are arguably more about a patient's individual values than medical treatments such as cardiac surgery or treatment for an infection.

Furthermore, critics of conscientious objection posit a distinction between the private and the public lives of medical professionals, according to which the *private*, deeply held views of clinicians should not influence their *public* professional practice. The basic idea is that health professionals are free to hold whatever views they want in private but that their conduct in the public realm should be informed by law, professional standards and patient preferences. Thus, Udo Schuklenk writes:

> What we are denying is that professionals are entitled to subvert the objectives of the profession they voluntarily joined by prioritizing their private beliefs over the professional delivery of services to the public, especially when they are monopoly purveyors of those services.
>
> (2016, 229)

Schuklenk does not wish to "deny anyone the right to hold any number of private religious or moral beliefs, as they see fit and as they choose to hold" (ibid.). He argues, however, that healthcare professionals who have a monopoly on the provision of a particular medical service should not refuse to provide that service to patients who are legally entitled to receive it (cf. LaFollette and LaFollette 2007).

3. A critique of contemporary models of medical practice

The foregoing discussion should suffice as an overview of the case against conscientious objection as it is presented in the bioethics literature. In this brief section I would like to raise a series of objections to the models of medicine just presented. Each of the models distorts in some way the role of healthcare practitioners.

Provider of services model of medicine

There are several serious problems with a PSM.[9] First, PSM leads to a steady erosion of professional authority. If indeed doctors are service providers, they should provide services as requested by patients (assuming that such services are within the scope of the law and professional guidelines). Individual practitioner discretion on ethical questions has no place in this model of medicine. The emphasis, rather, is on ensuring the reliability of service provision and satisfaction of consumer preferences. Such a paradigm inadvertently creates a tension between a doctor's exercise of clinical judgement and the preferences of patients. If indeed we place ultimate emphasis on preference satisfaction, then it seems that a doctor should provide services even when he or she deems such services to be in conflict with his or her understanding of the nature of medicine.

Second, PSM effectively hollows out traditional models of medical professionalism and replaces them with a government and market-focused account of medical practice. In the words of Curlin and Tollefsen, PSM's "pretense of moral seriousness is a charade and its attempts at professionalism are a facade" (2021, 3). Professionalism implies that practitioners interiorise medical norms and make an effort to practise the virtues constitutive of excellence in medicine. If you are told to be a mere service provider, however, it is unlikely that you will attempt to "make your own" the norms of medical practice. Rather, you will seek to *comply* with the norms of medicine as they are presented to you. Yet this is precisely what PSM encourages clinicians to do. It fosters an ethics of compliance in medicine rather than focusing on the virtue and character of clinicians.

Third, and most relevant to our purposes, the PSM sets up a conflict between the exercise of conscience and the fundamental, but minimal, norms of the profession. As the later chapters of this book suggest, conscience is an integral part of medical decision-making and the delivery of medical care. Rather than portraying conscience as an essential feature of good medical practice, PSM leads one to view the exercise of conscience with suspicion and as something that brings "private" and "personal" concerns to bear on transactions that should be governed by a physician's professional commitment to provide legally permitted services to patients who request these services. Conscience thus comes to be characterised as something extrinsic to medical practice rather than being something essential to good clinical judgement.

While conscience is marginalised by PSM, clinical practices which might ordinarily be seen as existing on the periphery of medicine (for example, euthanasia or cosmetic surgery) come be to accorded equal significance to procedures that we might consider to be at the centre of medicine (for example, cancer treatments or treatment for infectious diseases). The normative status of a medical procedure is determined by the law and by patient preferences. It is irrelevant that some clinical interventions do not appear to have therapeutic value or benefit for the patient (such extreme forms of cosmetic surgery for aesthetic purposes). What matters, rather, is whether a service is desired by patients and sanctioned by law and relevant professional associations. All procedures that fall within this ambit are on an equal ethical footing.

This approach is highly problematic. As Gamble and Pruski (2019) observe, a plausible distinction can be drawn between *medical acts* such as the treatment of a physical injury and what we might call *socio-clinical acts* such as abortion or euthanasia. The former might be defined as acts directed towards their patients' health whereas the latter might be defined as acts focused merely on the satisfaction of consumer wants (even if they necessarily involve some degree of clinical skill, which is the case with abortion). It seems fair to say that doctors can be expected to provide medical services that are necessary for the health of a patient.

It seems a stretch to say that doctors are obliged to provide all safe and legal socio-clinical services requested by patients. Indeed, this distinction is central to many arguments about the legitimate scope of conscientious objection. Several authors argue that doctors need not be expected to provide procedures that are peripheral to medical practice and fundamentally non-therapeutic in nature.

The "physicians, not conscripts" view

As we have seen, the "physicians, not conscripts" view claims that there is a tacit (or sometimes explicit) contract between service providers and the state according to which healthcare practitioners ought to provide services in accord with state expectations and patient preferences. At the very least, doctors "know what they are getting into" when they become members of the medical profession. Yet this account of clinician licensing and the "assumptions" that form part of one's entry into the medical profession is highly contentious. For one, admission to the medical profession does not involve a commitment to provide all medical services that are legal and sanctioned by the profession. *No such agreement exists*. With this in mind, a palliative care physician is not somehow violating their professional commitments by choosing not to participate in the provision of euthanasia or assisted suicide. Rather, the physician is legitimately exercising their professional freedom by refraining from participation in a service to which they have moral objection (let's assume, for argument's sake, that their objection will not have a disproportionate impact on patient access to that service). In any case, proponents of the "physicians, not conscripts" view do not do enough to justify why their particular interpretation of the tacit assumptions implicit in joining the medical profession is in fact the assumptions that are in play for all medical professionals. More work is needed to fill out the claim about the various expectations supposedly in play when doctors join the medical profession.

The fiduciary model

The fiduciary model does not command wide acceptance in the literature and for good reason. The principal problem with the fiduciary model is that it takes an account of professional ethics that is applied in professions such as law, and it attempts to impose this model onto medicine. In doing so, proponents of the fiduciary model fail to take account of the unique features of medicine as a profession that make it deserving of its own professional ethical framework. Medicine is a more complex and multifaceted enterprise than legal advocacy. True, a doctor ought to be a kind of advocate for a patient in the medical system. Yet it is also true that a doctor needs to guide a patient in their medical decision-making by presenting them with clinically indicated options and also providing a good account of their views on whether those options are indeed worth pursuing. We should also remember that there are ineradicable value assumptions built into medicine and that doctors cannot but make value judgements about particular practices. As such, the idea of a doctor suspending their own values and becoming a mere instrument for the fulfilment of patient preferences is unrealistic and ignores the ethical complexities of medicine. It would be wrong for a doctor to abrogate their ethical responsibilities under the guise of satisfying patient preferences. Doctors need to exercise their own capacities for ethical discernment to ensure that the way that they practise medicine is not only conducive to meeting patient needs but also in accord with good medical ethics. Contrary to the opinion of some ethicists, these two desiderata are not necessarily the same thing.

4. The case for re-examining the role of conscience in moral and professional life

This will suffice as an overview of the weaknesses of the case against conscientious objection. I do not purport to have addressed every argument against conscientious objection raised in the literature, but I do hope to have covered what I take to be the core assumptions underpinning the case against conscientious objection. One common claim made by critics is that one's duties to one's patients ought to take priority over personal integrity. McLeod, for example, writes that

> prioritizing [the moral integrity of physicians] over patients' interests – and therefore having unrestricted conscientious objection in healthcare – is seriously problematic . . . we would almost certainly be allowing harm . . . to patients.
>
> (2020, 115–116)

In this brief section, however, I will outline the case for revisiting our understanding of conscience and giving due importance to respecting the discretionary judgements of physicians. To be clear, I will not argue for unrestricted conscientious objection, but I will certainly argue for a broader right to conscientious objection than what critics have in mind.

Many arguments against conscientious objection rest on a fundamental misunderstanding of conscience and its role in moral and professional life. We need to develop a more detailed and philosophically rigorous account of conscience if we are to adequately understand its function in human moral psychology. Conscience, I will argue, is the aspect of human moral psychology that underpins an agent's personal engagement with morality. It leads one to engage at the deepest level possible with morality and its requirements. We ought also to consider the role that conscience plays in informing the moral and technical rationality of medical professionals. In the next two chapters, we will look extensively at the problems with the views on conscience and medicine outlined in the earlier sections of this chapter. I will argue that the faculty of conscience plays a much more significant role in the lives of physicians than many critics of conscientious objection would recognise. Medicine should not be reduced to a form of service delivery. On the contrary, medicine has a goal-directed character, and the goals at which medicine aims ought to inform our understanding of the norms of medical decision-making. Conscience is integral to discerning how to realise the medical good in particular situations.

Some critics of conscientious objection would readily acknowledge that conscience plays an important role in professional decision-making (Savulescu 2006; Kennett 2017). They may readily take on board the idea that conscience is a crucial part of decision-making in morally charged contexts, yet they may challenge the view that conscience ought to guide physician decision-making when it comes to safe and legal medical practices that are in accord with good ethics and that are desired by a patient. It could be argued patient preferences are a limiting principle on professional discretion. Provided that a patient is requesting services that are permitted under law and in accord with existing professional guidelines, a doctor ought to give a patient what they want.

This view is inconsistent. To claim that conscience is relevant to moral decision-making while denying its indispensable role in clinical judgements about controversial treatments is to draw an arbitrary distinction between situations in which conscience matters and situations in which it does not. Specifically, critics of conscientious objection posit an arbitrary dichotomy between *technical* and *moral* judgements in medicine. They presuppose that we can distinguish between matters in medicine that are of a technical nature and on which physicians should be able to exercise their discretionary judgement, and matters of a moral nature where physicians should defer to patients (Kinghorn 2013). The reality, however, is that we cannot distinguish technical and moral matters because they are ultimately two dimensions of the same clinical reality (Kinghorn 2013). While some contemporary philosophers might contend that the domains of science and ethics are entirely separate, the lived experience of professionals is such that facts and values are inextricably linked, and both come into play in clinical decision-making. Indeed, even the most banal decisions in medicine are directed at some good, be it health or the relief of suffering or even just human solidarity. As such, these decisions have an ethical dimension.

A physician acting on the basis of a considered understanding of medical practice, therefore, ought to be allowed to follow their conscience and refuse a procedure independent of whether their views accord with those of the medical establishment or whether they are minority opinions. Physicians ought to be able to follow their considered judgements provided they have consulted with their peers, have considered the best interests and preferences of patients and have identified principled reasons, within the bounds of reasonableness, for their chosen course of action.[10]

Critics of conscientious objection often unrealistically expect that clinicians ought to separate their private, personal and subjective values from their actions in the public realm of medicine (Savulescu 2006, 297). There seems to be a working assumption in the literature that one can psychologically compartmentalise one's life in such a way that one can stay true to one's deeply held commitments while simultaneously acting in a manner consonant with public neutrality and a rigid conception of the professional responsibilities of doctors. I will argue, however, that this expectation is psychologically unrealistic and that we should not expect doctors to set aside their personal beliefs in their public roles. Any attempt to do so threatens the moral agency and professional integrity of clinicians. With these considerations in mind, it is apposite to reconsider the moral weight that we place on conscience as a moral psychological faculty. Conscience is deserving of significantly more attention in moral philosophy and bioethics than it has received to date.

Conclusion

In this chapter I have explored the theoretical underpinnings of arguments against conscientious objection in medicine. In Section 1, I offered an overview of PSM and considered how an understanding of medicine as a form of service provision and a branch of the public service influences one's understanding of the moral responsibilities of doctors. I also discussed the fiduciary conception of medical practice defended by McLeod (2020). In Section 2, I discussed the implications that these views of medicine have for our understanding of the permissibility of conscientious objection. Critics argue that a physician's professional duty takes priority over his or her subjective values. Doctors should as a rule defer to patient preferences and the expectations of their employer and the profession when determining which medical treatments to provide. In Section 3, I identified a series of shortcomings of the case against conscientious objection. Critics of conscientious objection view conscience as being largely irrelevant to the practice of medicine. In Section 4, however, I argued that we ought to develop a more detailed and philosophically rigorous account of conscience if we are to adequately understand its function in human moral psychology and in the moral and technical rationality of medical professionals.

In the next chapter, I will offer a more detailed account of the role of conscience and will explore its role in the constitution of moral rationality and character. This will set the scene for Chapter 4, where I will look more specifically at the role of conscience in medical practice and how it ought to guide normative decision-making in the practice of medicine.

Notes

1 For a critique of the supposed objectivity of the notion of best interests in medicine, see the judgement of Brennan J. in *Marion's Case* [1992] HCA 15; (1992) 175 CLR 218.
2 See, for example, Wilkinson, Truog and Savulescu's (2016) defence of dissensus and individual practitioner discretion in end-of-life care.
3 I am not making a comment on the morality of contraception or the social benefits/ costs of contraception. My contention is that in this case contraceptives ought not to be construed as having a prophylactic purpose but rather have been prescribed for the purpose of providing a patient with sexual autonomy.
4 Note that the term 'conscientious objection' in English law has its origins in opposition to vaccination and not opposition to compulsory military service. See Robert M. Wolfe and Lisa K. Sharpe. "Antivaccinationists past and present". *British Medical Journal* 325 (2002): 430. It is not clear if Stahl and Emanuel are aware of this. That being said,

the practice of principled non-cooperation with state orders has a rich historical pedigree. This historical pedigree includes the practice of military conscription in modern nation states.

5 I prefer the language of "patient needs" to "patient interests" and "health interests". Needs, in my view, refer to the exigencies of human health whereas interests can refer to anything that a patient desires or wants regardless of whether it is conducive to his or her health. The former is more objective and desire-independent than the latter. This is not to deny the importance of a patient's subjective wishes in situations such as end-of-life care where a patient's personal values become increasingly important.

6 McLeod differs with scholars like Pellegrino who argued that the autonomy of patients and the autonomy of physicians must *both* be respected: "The physician-patient relationship, like any ethical relationship, is a reciprocal one. In the justifiable concern for patient autonomy, it is easy to forget that the physician is a moral agent as well as the patient. As such, the physician's autonomy, as well as the patient's, is deserving of respect. When the two are in conflict, the patient's wish does not automatically trump the physician's." See Edmund Pellegrino. "Patient and physician autonomy: Conflicting rights and obligations in the physician-patient relationship". *Journal of Contemporary Health Law and Policy* 10;47 (1994): 47–68.

7 It is worth noting that this criticism of conscientious objection was addressed in the previous chapter when we distinguished conscientious objection from a mere dislike of some aspect of one's professional responsibilities.

8 For a critique of Giubilini and Savulescu's view, see Michal Pruski. "Reply to: Beyond money: Conscientious objection in medicine as a conflict of interests". *Journal of Bioethical Inquiry* 18;1 (2021): 177–180.

9 In this section I draw heavily on the work of Curlin and Tollefsen (2021).

10 We will discuss the criteria that make up a standard of reasonableness in Chapter 4.

References

Berlinger, Nancy. *Are Workarounds Ethical? Managing Moral Problems in Health Care Systems*. London: Oxford University Press, 2015.

Charo, Alta. "The celestial fire of conscience: Refusing to deliver medical care". *New England Journal of Medicine* 352 (2005): 2471–2473.

Cholbi, Michael. "Public cartels, private conscience". *Philosophy, Politics and Economics* 17;4 (2018): 356–377.

Clarke, Steve. "Conscientious objection in healthcare, referral and the military analogy". *Journal of Medical Ethics* 43 (2017): 218–221.

Cohen, Carl. "Conscientious objection". *Ethics* 78;4 (1968): 269–279.

Curlin, Farr, and Tollefsen, Christopher. *The Way of Medicine: Ethics and the Healing Profession*. South Bend: University of Notre Dame Press, 2021.

Earp, Brian. "Does religion deserve a place in secular medicine". *Journal of Medical Ethics* 41 (2015): 865–866.

Gamble, Nathan, and Pruski, Michal. "Medical acts and conscientious objection: What can a physician be compelled to do?". *The New Bioethics* 25 (2019): 262–282.

Giubilini, Alberto, and Savulescu, Julian. "Beyond money: Conscientious objection in medicine as a conflict of interest". *Journal of Bioethical Inquiry* 17 (2020): 229–243.

Hahn Chaet, Danielle. "The AMA code of medical ethics' opinions on patient decision-making capacity and competence and surrogate decision making". *AMA Journal of Ethics* 19;7 (2017): 675–677.

Hui, E.C. "Doctors as fiduciaries: A legal construct of the patient-physician relationship". *Hong Kong Medical Journal* 11;6 (2005): 527–529.

Kennett, Jennette. "Kant on conscience and conscientious objection". *Cambridge Quarterly of Healthcare Ethics* 26 (2017): 69–81.

Kilbride, Madison, and Joffe, Stephen. "The new age of patient autonomy: Implications for the physician-patient relationship". *JAMA* 320 (2018): 1973–1974.

Kim, Andrew Chongseh. "When the apocalypse comes, will anything change: Gay marriage, black lives matter, and the rule of law". *Savannah Law Review* 3;1 (2016): 57–77.

Kinghorn, Warren. "Conscience as clinical judgment: Medical education and the virtue of prudence". *Virtual Mentor* 15;3 (2013): 202–205.

LaFollette, Eva, and LaFollette, Hugh. "Private conscience, public acts". *Journal of Medical Ethics* 33 (2007): 249–254.

Lysaught, Therese. "Respect, or how respect for persons became respect for autonomy". *Journal of Medicine and Philosophy* 29;6 (2004): 665–680.

McLeod, Carolyn. *Conscience in Reproductive Health Care: Prioritizing Patient Interests*. London: Oxford University Press, 2020.

Mehlman, Maxwell J. "Why physicians are fiduciaries for their patients". *Indiana Health Law Review* 12;1 (2015): 1–63.

Omelianchuk, Adam. "Do you have a 'syndrome' if you have a flat shaped head". *Journal of Medicine and Philosophy* 43;4 (2018): 369–380.

Parker, Malcolm, Wardle, Jon, Weir, Malcolm, and Stewart, Cameron. "Medical merchants: Conflict of interest, office product sales and notifiable conduct". *Medical Journal of Australia* 194;1 (2011): 34–37.

Pellegrino, Edmund D. "Patient and physician autonomy: Conflicting rights and obligations in the physician-patient relationship". *Journal of Contemporary Health Law and Policy* 10;47 (1994): 47–68.

Pellegrino, Edmund D. "Philosophy of medicine and medical ethics: A phenomenological perspective". In George Khushf (ed.). *Handbook of Bioethics: Taking Stock of the Field from a Philosophical Perspective*. Dordrecht: Kluwer, 2004: 183–202.

Raley, Bill. "How conscientious objectors killed the draft: The collapse of the selective service during the Vietnam War". *Cleveland State Law Review* 68;2 (2020): 151–171.

Rousseau, Jean Jacques. *Emile: Or On Education*. Barbara Foxley (trans.). London & Toronto: J.M. Dent and Sons, 1921 [1762].

Savulescu, Julian. "Conscientious objection in medicine". *British Medical Journal* 332 (2006): 294–297.

Savulescu, Julian, and Schuklenk, Udo. "Doctors have no right to refuse medical assistance in dying, abortion or contraception". *Bioethics* 31;3 (2017): 162–170.

Schuklenk, Udo. "Accommodating conscientious objection in medicine: Private ideological convictions must not trump professional obligations". *Journal of Clinical Ethics* 27;3 (2016): 227–232.

Schuklenk, Udo, and Smalling, Ricardo. "Why medical professionals have no moral claim to conscientious objection accommodation in liberal democracies". *Journal of Medical Ethics* 43 (2017): 234–240.

Stahl, Ronit, and Emanuel, Ezekiel. "Physicians not conscripts; conscientious objection in healthcare". *The New England Journal of Medicine* 376;14 (2017): 1380–1385.

Sulmasy, Daniel. "Tolerance, professional judgement, and the discretionary space of the physician". *Cambridge Quarterly of Healthcare Ethics* 21;6 (2017): 18–31.

Symons, Xavier. "Conscientious objection: Why the professional duty argument is unconvincing". *Journal of Medicine and Philosophy* forthcoming.

Tollefsen, Christopher, and Curlin, Farr. "Conscience and the way of medicine". *Perspectives on Medicine and Biology* 62;3 (2019): 560–575.

Tollefsen, Christopher, and Curlin, Farr. *The Way of Medicine: Ethics and the Healing Profession*. South Bend: Notre Dame University Press, 2021.

United Kingdom Parliament. "Conscription: The first world war". London: UK Parliament, 2021. Available from www.parliament.uk/about/living-heritage/transformingsociety/private-lives/yourcountry/overview/conscription/

Walzer, Michael. *Just and Unjust Wars: A Moral Argument With Historical Illustrations* (2nd ed.). New York: Basic Books, 1992.

Wilkinson, Dominic, Truog, Robert, and Savulescu, Julian. "In favour of dissensus: Why we should agree to disagree about end-of-life decisions". *Bioethics* 30;2 (2016): 109–118.

Wolfe, Robert M., and Sharpe, Lisa K. "Antivaccinationists past and present". *British Medical Journal* 325 (2002): 430.

3 A theory of conscience – part I
Conscience and moral life

Introduction

The aim of this chapter and the next is to provide clarity on how conscience is relevant to moral and political debates and, in particular, how a robust conception of conscience might inform our understanding of conscientious objection in medicine. In this chapter, I offer an account of the role of conscience in human moral psychology and also consider why restrictions on conscience do grave harm to moral agents. This chapter provides the moral psychological backdrop for Chapter 4, in which I discuss the role that conscience plays in guiding ethical deliberation in medical practice.

My focus in this chapter is what one might call a *well-developed conscience*. It is true that someone might have a conscience that has been poorly formed, depleted or suppressed such that they may deceive themselves about their actions/intentions/desires or be unaware of their responsibilities and obligations. Indeed, the spectre of a morally compromised doctor with a toxic conscience is one of the main concerns associated with permitting the exercise of conscience in medicine. For the most part, however, the content of this chapter presupposes a conscience that is well formed and well functioning.

This chapter will primarily consider how conscience informs an agent's outlook on morality. Yet conscience is sometimes described as a source of religious insight and as a monitor of fidelity in general, not just moral fidelity (Langston 2001; Velleman 2009, 104–105). While I will focus on the role that conscience plays in motivating us to live a moral life, the boundary between the moral life and other aspects of an agent's life is vague, and this should be borne in mind as we discuss the notion of fundamental beliefs and commitments. I suspect that many aspects of life have or can have a moral dimension if only we think carefully or broadly enough to recognise that moral dimension. Various philosophers, for example, have written lucidly on the relationship between art and morality, and it would be eminently reasonable for an artist to speak of their professional work as having a moral dimension (Keiran 2003). With this idea in mind, I think that an agent's deep commitments, even if they do not fall within the ambit of our intuitive notions of morality, are still relevant when thinking through the moral importance of respect for conscience.

DOI: 10.4324/9781003247623-3

Section 1 of this chapter considers how we might conceptualise the role of conscience in human moral psychology. I argue that conscience provides us with an awareness of the personal nature of moral obligation. That is, conscience leads agents to view morality in relation to their own self and character and to commit to living up to the requirements of the moral life. In Section 2, I consider how human beings are harmed when the exercise of conscience is restricted. Some theorists note that violations of conscience can lead to severe emotional trauma. Yet I want to focus instead on the implications that the suppression of conscience has for one's character and one's self. Restrictions on the exercise of conscience, I contend, prevent agents from living in accord with their own considered understanding of the requirements of morality. Related to this, they subvert an agent's pursuit of life projects that give one meaning and purpose. Finally, they undermine features of moral rationality that are prerequisite of agency.

1. The role of conscience in human moral psychology

Conscience gives human beings an awareness of their moral duties and facilitates moral reflection. Few would disagree with this. Where disagreement arises is in explaining *how* conscience yields moral awareness. With this in mind, I will argue that conscience gives agents an *existential awareness of their moral obligations*. This is in contrast to a view that supposes that conscience gives us direct, intuitive and substantive knowledge about the rightness and wrongness of particular acts. Rather than being a source of direct moral knowledge, I will describe conscience as a meta-capacity underpinning a moral agent's commitment to acting in accord with what they judge to be right and good. Conscience is above all a commitment to doing what one knows to be right. Related to this, I will argue that conscience monitors the coherence between an agent's self-identifying beliefs and intentions and their practical actions (D'Arcy 1961; Blustein 1993; Benjamin 1995; Velleman 2009; Wicclair 2011; McLeod 2020). Subsection named "Conscience as a source of moral fidelity rather than intuitive moral knowledge" will discuss how conscience gives moral agents an existential awareness of their moral obligations. In the subsection titled "Conscience as a source of moral awareness", I will briefly discuss the relationship between conscience and emotions. This will prepare us for a discussion in Section 2 of the moral harm that agents sustain when they violate their conscience.

Conscience as a source of moral fidelity rather than intuitive moral knowledge

In this subsection, I argue that conscience provides agents with an existential awareness of their moral obligations. I critically evaluate different ways in which conscience can be said to provide moral knowledge and argue that conscience yields an awareness of the personal relevance of moral obligation rather than providing substantive knowledge about the rightness or wrongness of actions. In doing so, I depart from a long tradition of theorising about conscience that dates back to at least the early modern period.

There are countless ancient and modern philosophers who discussed the idea of conscience whom I will not mention. Rather, the following discussion focuses on those philosophers who have been the most notable proponents of an intuitionist account of conscience (the account of conscience that I believe is quite common in the literature today and that is thus necessary to critique). Suffice to say that there are several traditions of theorising on conscience that are not discussed in this subsection as comprehensive discussion of the history of conscience is not possible here.

A moral intuitionist account of conscience

Several early modern philosophers argued that conscience is a source of moral knowledge and plays an integral role in giving agents epistemic access to moral facts (Shaftesbury 1999/1711; Hume 1975/1740; Rousseau 1921/1762). Importantly, what we are referring to here is *not* the role that conscience plays in motivating agents to deliberate about how they ought to act. Rather, the claim is that conscience gives agents an intuitive grasp of the content of morality. That is to say, conscience gives us particular knowledge of the rightness or wrongness of actions. Conscience, in this regard, is not a stimulus for obtaining moral knowledge but is actually a source of moral knowledge itself.

The meaning of the term "moral knowledge" is indeterminate, however, and we must clarify what kind of moral knowledge conscience can be said to provide. Conscience is sometimes portrayed as a homunculus that whispers ethical guidance in the ears of moral agents. The commonly used metaphor of conscience as a "voice" is an example of this homuncular view of conscience (Schinkel 2007, 117–121). It is tempting, based on this caricature, to suggest that conscience gives us an intuitive grasp of moral truth. One might be inclined to describe conscience as "a distinct mental faculty, an intuitive moral sense that determines the rightness and wrongness of actions" (Sulmasy 2008, 136).[1] Rousseau was a proponent of this view and described conscience as "an innate principle of justice and virtue, by which . . . we judge our own actions or those of others to be good or evil" (Rousseau 1762/1921, 253). According to Rousseau, conscience frees us from "childish errors" and the "prejudices of our upbringing" and provides a "true guide" for virtuous action (Rousseau 1762/1921, 252–253). Conscience, in this sense, provides us with a clear and unadulterated view of the requirements of virtue and justice.

Conscience might also be described as a faculty deep in our psyche that we must "search" to discover what the right thing is to do. At the surface of our moral psychology, we may find many conflicting ideas that characterise our moral reasoning – ideas that are the products of cultural, religious or political conditioning. Introspection or soul searching is required to get at the content of conscience, which in turn gives us a window into the content of morality. Bishop Butler, for example, described conscience as a faculty of the mind that "pronounces determinately some actions to be in themselves evil, wrong, unjust" (Butler 1726/1950:

Sermon II). One might think that we discern moral truth by making ourselves more attentive to these pronouncements of conscience deep in our consciousness.

Yet the intuitionist account of conscience does not seem right as conscience can often lead people to adopt manifestly immoral beliefs. If conscience provided knowledge of the substantive content of morality – if it were a special sensibility deep in our consciousness that gave us epistemic access to particular moral facts – then all moral reasoning could be concluded with the recommendation that each moral agent should "follow their conscience" (Ojakangas 2013). Rather than engaging in moral reflection and dialogue to determine how one should act in particular situations, one could follow the quiet voice echoing in the depth of one's heart and use this as a moral guide. Yet experience indicates that the inner voice of conscience can be seriously misguided. Someone might, for example, have racist intuitions and may sincerely believe that some races are superior to others. Other agents might have discriminatory intuitions about matters of gender, religion, class and so on. Conscience defined as a source of moral intuition, in this respect, is neither infallible nor even reliable. Rather, in some cases it reflects a perverse moral logic.

Even if conscience of this sort were in and of itself reliable, agents would still face practical problems in trying to discern what guidance conscience is providing to them. The voice of conscience could be drowned out or mimicked by other features of our moral psychology. As Hill (1998) writes:

> Whether or not we believe that conscience itself is infallible, we must still acknowledge that we can make mistakes about whether what we take to be dictates of conscience are authentic. Wishful thinking, fear, childhood prejudices, and indoctrination in false ideologies can imitate or distort the voice of conscience, especially if we have dulled that voice by frequently disregarding it. So in effect, the doctrine that conscience is very reliable, even infallible, with regard to objective right and wrong is subject to practical qualifications.

The issue is not just that conscience can itself err and lead moral agents astray. Even if conscience in and of itself is reliable, agents can still face practical problems in trying to discern what guidance conscience is providing to them. What we might think is the voice of conscience may in fact be some prejudice that we have acquired in childhood or from the cultural or professional milieu in which we are immersed.

There are significant problems, therefore, in describing conscience as a source of intuitive knowledge about the rightness or wrongness of particular acts. I do not want to completely disregard this view of conscience, as I do think there is merit to the idea that one must form one's conscience for it to function as a reliable source of moral knowledge (O'Shea 2018). That is to say, I believe that we can educate our own moral sensibilities in ways that will conform them more with moral truth. We can, for example, interrogate our intuitions in the light of widely accepted political or religious principles (such as a commitment to human rights or to the common good) and thus ensure that our intuitions are reliable. This qualification might help to rescue the intuitionist view from some of the powerful objections that it faces.

Furthermore, I think there is merit to the idea that conscience is, in one sense of the word, concerned with an application of general moral knowledge to particular moral facts. Saad, for example, defines conscience as "an act of reasoning whereby a general moral principle is applied to a specific situation in order to generate a judgement about how one should or should not act" (2019, 253). This is equivalent to a traditional account of conscience along the lines of what Thomas Aquinas had in mind when he discussed conscience (Hoffmann 2012). Indeed, this is quite different from an intuitionist account of conscience, as it involves reasoning about how general moral principles apply to particular cases rather than a kind of mental illumination whereby one spontaneously apprehends what the right course of action is.

Yet precisely for this reason, it is not wise to focus on an *intuitionist* account of conscience – at least insofar as we are trying to make the case for ensuring that conscience is respected in law and professional codes of conduct. The intuitionist account of conscience raises too many concerns about the fallibility of our own moral compass and the inscrutable psychological origins of moral intuition. If we want to make the case for respecting consciences, we should be wary of conceptualising conscience as a source of intuitive knowledge of the substantive content of morality.

Conscience as a source of moral awareness

The moral potential of conscience, however, is not limited to intuitive knowledge about the rightness or wrongness of particular acts. Conscience, rather, can be said to yield a conviction that one ought to act in accord with the demands of morality. Note that an agent can have general moral knowledge without that knowledge engaging them at a personal level and leading them to change their behaviour. A teenager may, for example, believe that theft is wrong in the abstract without really believing that they should refrain from engaging in acts of petty theft from the supermarket. Or a computer programmer may believe that theft is wrong without feeling moved to refrain from unlawfully using others' intellectual property. Moral knowledge, in these cases, does not move an agent to act morally. Someone may, therefore, know something at a cognitive level (e.g. that theft is wrong) without this leading them to refrain from immoral actions (e.g. particular acts of theft).

Several philosophers (Fuss 1964; Blustein 1993; Sulmasy 2008) have argued that conscience is precisely that feature of our moral psychology that gives us a "a felt conviction" that we ought to do what we know to be right and good. That is, conscience provides an agent with the concrete, existential conviction that we ought to carry out those kinds of actions that practical reason has deemed to be morally obligatory.[2] As Fuss writes, "conscience affords one the 'existential knowledge' (more properly, the existential conviction) that he is under obligation to do what he knows to be right and to pursue what he judges to be good"

(1964, 116). Similarly, Blustein writes that "conscience indicates a particular way of seeing moral and other normative demands, a mode of consciousness in which prospective actions are viewed in relation to one's self and character" (Blustein 1993, 294). What we are describing here is not a substantive belief arising from practical reason, nor even a process of inference from general to particular moral knowledge. Rather, conscience in this sense is better described as yielding a deep belief at the core of one's being that "one must act in accordance with what he knows or believes [to be right]" (Fuss 1964, 116). Conscience is a meta-ethical awareness about how one ought to respond to the moral insights provided by practical reason as well as the beliefs that form the content of one's character. This is different from the substantive knowledge that people typically associate with conscience. But conscience as a source of conviction is just as important, if not more important than conscience, as an act of moral judgement.

Conscience, according to this view, gives agents an awareness that they have a personal stake in pursuing a moral life. This existential awareness provided by conscience leads one to make a commitment to conscientiously observing the requirements of morality. Thus, Sulmasy (2008, 138) writes:

> [Conscience involves] a commitment to uphold one's deepest self-identifying moral beliefs; a commitment to discern the moral features of particular cases as best one can, and to reason morally to the best of one's ability; . . . a commitment to make decisions according to the best of one's moral ability and to act upon what one discerns to be the morally right course of action.

Conscience, in other words, leads us to be *conscientious* with respect to the demands of morality and moral life. It gives us an awareness that our flourishing as moral agents is tied up with living a moral life in a conscientious manner and seeking to discern the good in particular situations. Conscience leads agents to "assent to the truth that one should act morally" (Sulmasy 2008, 138).

Conscience – understood as a personal engagement with morality – does not necessarily track true moral knowledge. Conscience can, in some cases, be led astray by practical reason (Anscombe 2005, 238–241). It may be the case, for example, that a soldier forms the belief that the torture of innocent civilians is morally permissible. The soldier may feel a strong existential conviction, arising from conscience, that they are duty bound to carry out torture if they receive such an order from a commanding officer. Conscience, then, could be said to yield a conviction that the soldier should do what, in the last analysis, is morally impermissible. So we should resist the claim that conscience is an infallible moral guide, even if we do think it provides us with personal moral awareness. This is not to say that conscience itself goes awry – strictly speaking, it is practical reason that errs. That is to say, practical reason, not conscience, is the principle cause of mistakes in moral reasoning. But conscience is responsive to practical reason, and as such will be implicated in the errors of practical reason (Fuss 1964, 117).[3] Indeed, conscience can be deformed in various ways and must be educated if it is to function as a tracker of the moral good.

One of the practical functions of conscience, closely linked to its role in fostering a personal engagement with morality, is to ensure that there is coherence between our deep beliefs, our moral actions and the objective moral order. Conscience monitors the extent to which our practical actions cohere with those beliefs that form part of our moral character. Vice versa, conscience monitors the extent to which our deep beliefs cohere with our actions in the world. As Sulmasy (2008, 138) writes,

> The activity of conscience is a meta-judgment that arises in particular moral deliberations. It is a judgment that a proposed act (or an act one has already accomplished) would violate one's fundamental moral commitments, including, importantly, a fundamental moral commitment to act with understanding.

People can, of course, have different fundamental moral commitments. Conscience does not prescribe what sorts of commitments a person must have. But it does monitor the extent to which a person is living up to these commitments, whatever they may be, and it also monitors whether one is living in accord with one's understanding of morality and reality. Conscience is an advocate, so to speak, for a person's deepest beliefs and for reality as it is known by moral agents.

Conscience, then, tracks moral integrity. The *integrity view of conscience* has been widely defended in recent literature on conscience (Benjamin 1995, 470; Childress 1979, 322; Blustein 1993, 300; Sulmasy 2008, 138; Lyons 2009, 488–494). As stated earlier, proponents of this view argue that conscience is concerned with personal integrity understood in terms of inner, psychological unity. Inner unity is valuable, according to these authors, either because integrity contributes to our having a good life (Benjamin 1995, 470; Blustein 1993), or because unity and the desire to repair "inner division" are admirable characteristics of persons (Blustein 1993, 297). Conscience is a feature of our moral psychology that is responsible for preserving unity between our deeply held beliefs and our practical actions. It makes us alert to signs of discord between our actions or thoughts and our deep moral commitments, and it inclines us to assuage such discord.

Is it necessary to posit a level of moral awareness over and above practical reason? One might argue that practical reason alone is sufficient to explain why we feel compelled to follow our moral obligations and that we need not posit the existence of conscience to explain why people are committed to living a moral life. Conscience, on this picture, is redundant, at least when it comes to explaining why people live morally upright lives. Alternatively, one might argue that it is moral virtue, not conscience, that makes us responsive to moral reasons. We might describe virtues as the underlying dispositions that make agents responsive to the right kinds of moral reasons (Audi and Murphy 2006; Cullity 2017). That is to say, virtues are dispositions to act in the right way based on the right moral reasons. If indeed moral and intellectual virtues dispose an agent to respond appropriately to practical reason, then one might argue that it is unnecessary to posit the existence of a moral sensibility like conscience whereby we become responsive to the imperatives of practical reason.

The trouble with these alternative perspectives, however, is that they focus on our responsiveness to specific moral reasons rather than the existential conviction that one ought to live a moral life. Practical reason tells us what the good is, or what the correct course of action is, and virtue disposes us to act based on the right moral reasons. But neither practical reason nor virtues explains why we are personally invested in morality or that we feel that the moral life matters in earnest. Practical reason may very well yield specific moral knowledge in the form of normative propositions about the world. But this does not give an agent the conviction that they ought to act on this knowledge. Virtue may make us responsive to the right moral reasons, but it does not explain why an agent makes a fundamental commitment to living a moral life. Conscience is precisely that aspect of our moral psychology that yields a personal sense of moral obligation. It is that feature of psychology whereby an agent recognises that he is "under obligation to do what he knows to be right and to pursue what he judges to be good" (Fuss 1964, 116). Indeed, perhaps the best way to describe conscience here is as the kind of cognitive capacity that is absent in a psychopath. A psychopath lacks the kinds of sentiments – empathy, compassion, guilt and remorse – that underpin a personal commitment to act morally.

One might argue that one reason why practical reason is *practical* is that it prompts action. The problem with this view is that there are many examples where a moral agent knows what the right thing is to do and yet does not do it. We need to invoke other moral concepts to explain what leads agents to act in accord with the ordinances of practical reason. Virtue provides part of this explanation insofar as it makes us responsive to the right kinds of moral reasons. But virtue does not explain the more basic fact that moral agents feel compelled to live up to the precepts of morality. That is to say, virtue does not explain why an agent comprehends morality as something in which his very character is implicated. To put it another way: virtue may lead agents to love *the good*, but virtue builds upon a more fundamental realisation that *the good* is not just an abstract concept but rather the good of one's self and character. This latter realisation is the role of conscience that I am primarily focused on in this book.

This is one significant way that my account of conscience differs from that offered by philosopher Kimberley Brownlee in her 2012 book *Conscience and Conviction: The Case for Civil Disobedience*. Brownlee describes conscience as a principle of moral responsiveness in agents, and she links the cultivation of conscience to the cultivation of practical wisdom, virtue and objective moral integrity. Yet it seems that at least some of the descriptions that Brownlee provides of conscience – such as when she describes conscience as "a set of practical moral skills" (52) and "a guide to good conduct" (54) – make conscience sound a lot like practical reason or virtue. This approach runs the risk of rendering conscience redundant in our explanation of human moral psychology. It is this accusation of redundancy that I wish to avoid by describing conscience as *meta-capacity* which makes an agent aware of his or her personal investment in living a moral life. Granted, Brownlee also describes conscience "as a sustained commitment to improving ourselves as moral beings" (55), which makes her account sound much more like a meta-capacity. But she also at times appears to conflate conscience with lower-order moral psychological functions, and I am inclined to reject these aspects of her theory.

This should suffice as a first approximation of my understanding of the role of conscience in human moral psychology. Importantly, I do not want to overstate the originality of my account of conscience. Ultimately, the position I am advancing is a close cousin of the view advanced by Brownlee and very similar to the view advanced by Sulmasy (2008). At this juncture it is instructive to take a closer look at the relationship between conscience and the emotions before considering in greater detail how restrictions on the exercise of conscience affect character and the self.

Conscience and the emotions

Conscience is often described as "pricking" and "prodding" moral agents so that they follow their better moral judgement (Wood 2008). John Cottingham, for example, writes that

> it appears to be part of the concept of conscience that it involves not just the evaluation of one's past conduct, but also, when the evaluation is negative, a characteristic sense of discomfort.
>
> (Cottingham 2013, 733)

In this brief section I will discuss the moral emotions associated with conscience such as anxiety, guilt, shame and remorse. I will argue that emotions are the way in which conscience makes its operations felt by an agent but that we should be careful not to conflate moral emotions with the operations of conscience.

Based on a superficial analysis, we might be tempted to claim that the emotions are a constituent feature of conscience and that moral emotions such as guilt and shame *just are* what it means to have a conscience. Yet this is incorrect. While emotions are closely associated with conscience, conscience is not, strictly speaking, a sentiment or an affection. As Sulmasy writes:

> The exercise of conscience is . . . accompanied by emotions such as satisfaction or guilt. . ., but the act of conscience itself is a meta-moral judgment, not an emotion.
>
> (Sulmasy 2008, 138)

The basic point is that conscience is not equivalent to the emotions, even though it triggers certain emotional reactions. Rather, conscience yields an existential awareness of our moral responsibilities, which takes the form of either an act of the will – in the form of an assent to the truth that one should act morally – or an act of judgement – whereby we discern whether an act is in accord with our fundamental moral commitments (Sulmasy 2008, 138). Emotions may arise as a result of judgements of conscience, yet they are not equivalent with the operations of conscience. As Stoker (2018) writes:

> a phenomenon without any [or with only insignificant] emotional stirrings . . . could hardly be a phenomenon of conscience. . . . But [one that] viewed [urgings] as no more than subjective feelings. . . [w]ould have to be blind to the essence of conscience.

Emotions like guilt and shame should rather be thought of as the way in which conscience makes an agent aware of its operations and exerts influence on an agent. We might think of so-called *moral emotions*, then, as affective manifestations of the action of conscience, alerting an agent to the extent to which they are living up to the requirements of morality.

By invoking the notion of moral emotions, I do not wish to delve too deeply into a theory of the emotions, if only because this is not particularly relevant to our discussion. Nor do I wish to draw a strong distinction between supposedly moral emotions and other natural emotions. All I am claiming is that there is a subset of the emotions that human beings experience which are often best explained with reference to moral life. As Childress writes, "when an agent explains why he experiences certain feelings, he will sometimes offer a moral explanation". "Moral feelings", he argues, "are those feelings that are explained by moral notions" (1979, 322). Two examples are guilt and shame. According to Childress, guilt is often associated with a violation of some aspect of "society's basic morality, its stations, duties, and obligations". Shame, in contrast, is typically associated with "the morality of aspiration, ideals, and supererogation" (1979, 322–323).[4] Other moral emotions such as anxiety and remorse may also be relevant to conscience. Rather than discussing these emotions in detail, however, I shall simply observe that they are associated with a judgement that one has failed to live up to one's moral obligations – either those obligations that come to one from society or those obligations that agents impose on themselves.

At risk of stating the obvious, it is important to emphasise that moral agents have a strong aversion to the negative moral emotions associated with conscience. As Childress writes, the motivation that agents have for acting morally is "in part, avoidance of a sanction imposed by the self on itself" (1979, 328). Childress argues that "[w]hen a person appeals to his conscience" – when someone says that they cannot do something in good conscience – that individual indicates their "liability to certain feelings which [they predict] will result from acting in certain ways" (1979, 322). An agent does not want to be left with a "bad conscience" and on this basis will ask to be excused from participation in the said action. What we are talking about here is not just a feeling of mild psychological discomfort that someone might feel after acting in a particular way. Rather, a serious failure to act in accord with one's conscience is registered at all levels of our psychosomatic constitution. Thus, Lyons writes:

> [The censure of conscience] will be registered internally, not only in our conscious thoughts, but also as "bodily motions" . . . for emotions are complex psychosomatic episodes that involve not only our cognitive and evaluative attitudes but also our visceral reactions. . . [which] provide the feelings integral to the emotions.
>
> (2009, 493)

Lyons goes on to note that "our emotions are probably the truest manifestation of our deepest values, for the reason that we cannot easily dissemble in regard to them" (2009, 493). One cannot, in other words, just ignore the "pangs" of conscience.

Two additional observations are in order here. First, I am not attempting to reduce the emotional sanction of conscience to guilt and shame. Rather, the sanction of conscience can also take the form of experiences of emotional numbness and a sense of depersonalisation, whereby an agent becomes existentially disengaged from her life and actions. As we will discuss in the next section, an agent's identity is liable to dissolution when she fails to act with integrity, as the agent's deeply held beliefs may cease to have any real bearing on her practical actions. At the very least, there is a sense in which an agent's central beliefs and commitments (which form part of the content of identity) are weakened when she fails to act in accord with them. This weakening of one's personal identity can lead to feelings of depersonalisation, whereby agents experience a sense of alienation from themselves and the world they inhabit. Related to this, agents may experience emotional numbness, as they are not as personally engaged in the world as they would be if they were acting in accord with their own deeply held beliefs. To quote Nathaniel Hawthorne, "to the untrue man, the whole universe is false" (2007, 115). Someone who is unmoved by her own deeply held convictions is less likely to be moved by the moral plight of other human beings.

Second, there are parallel positive emotions that arise when one has acted in accord with one's conscience. A "clear conscience" is not just associated with an absence of moral torment. Rather, moral integrity is associated with deep feelings of peace, contentment, even joy. When one acts in accord with conscience, one may experience a palpable sense of the order and coherence in one's own psychology. Indeed, Aquinas described peace as the "tranquillity of order", and there is a very real sense in which peace – understood in this way – manifests itself in the psychology of someone who consistently acts in a manner reflective of their deeply held beliefs (Ramsay 1997). Obviously, someone who has morally perverse beliefs about the world may suffer from chronic psychological disturbance (it seems that integrity won't do much to allay the hatred and anger that a white supremacist harbours, for example). Yet presuming that an agent is not morally deranged, it is plausible to suggest that integrity will help bring a sense of peace to one's psychology.

In light of the relationship between conscience and emotions, some philosophers describe conscience as a principle of unity in human persons. Conscience is not just a purely rational faculty that makes us aware of our moral obligations. Rather, conscience also affects our emotional states and has the capacity to induce emotions such as guilt and shame as well as corresponding feelings of peace and contentment when we live up to our moral obligations. As Sulmasy writes, conscience "unifies the cognitive, conative, and emotional aspects of the moral life" (2008, 138). It is conscience that ensures that the content of our reflective moral judgements is mirrored by our emotions.

The connection between this portrayal of conscience and the notion of moral injury in military ethics cannot be overlooked. Moral injury refers to the "damage done to one's conscience or moral compass when that person perpetrates, witnesses or fails to prevent acts that transgress one's own moral beliefs, values or ethical codes of conduct" (Moral Injury Project 2014). The basic claim motivating the moral injury literature is that soldiers suffer some deep personal injury by being forced to kill civilians or conduct torture, or even if they kill civilians by accident, or just kill anyone. While there is debate about how to best define this notion, it is certainly the case that many soldiers experience post-service trauma as a result of being ordered to act in a manner contrary to their better moral judgement. This experience is not dissimilar to the "pangs" of conscience described in Debra Hanna's widely cited psychological study of nurses who have been compelled against their wishes to participate in elective abortions (Hanna 2005). Just as in the case of moral injury in war, someone who violates their conscience in some serious way (be it in a professional or social context or in private life) is liable to experience deep personal injury and indeed feelings of depersonalisation that typically characterise post-traumatic stress subsequent to deployment in a theatre of war.

If the case against conscientious objection in medicine were to succeed, critics would need to show how restrictions on the exercise of conscience in healthcare would not lead to moral injury, or, alternatively, they would need to justify regulations that inflict moral injury on healthcare practitioners. Neither of these claims would be easy to demonstrate. It is difficult to see how restrictions on the exercise of conscience would not lead to situations in which healthcare practitioners were forced to violate their consciences, leading to at least some form of moral injury. Moral injury of any kind, furthermore, is a very serious matter, and one would need strong countervailing reasons to justify the infliction of injury on healthcare practitioners. Claims about delays in access to abortion or limits on access to euthanasia or whatever service one is concerned about would need to be significantly bolstered if they are to justify the infliction of moral injury on healthcare practitioners.

2. The costliness of violating conscience

This section discusses the consequences of suppressing or restricting the exercise of conscience (whether this is done internally by an agent themselves or by external coercion). The emotional sanction of conscience is often thought to be the most significant harm of restrictions on conscientious objection. In this section, however, I will argue that moral agents risk losing their basic orienting ideals if they act in a manner contrary to their conscience. Repeated and serious violations of conscience imperil one's basic values and one's sense of meaning and purpose. Agents who abandon their deeply held beliefs and commitments, furthermore, also undermine their capacity for independent moral judgement. Our personal moral ideals are an epistemic standpoint from which we can independently judge the social and professional norms of the communities to which we belong. This has implications for moral agency. To the extent that one lacks personal moral ideals, or one allows these ideals to be eroded, one loses the capacity for judging and acting independently of the norms underpinning the social practices of which one is a part.

It is appropriate to begin with a consideration of how different theorists conceptualise so-called *appeals to conscience*. Some theorists trivialise the function of conscience in the moral life and suggest that the impact of contravening or suppressing conscience is negligible. These critics characterise appeals to conscience as mere expressions of likes or dislikes rather than associating these appeals with deeply held, identity-conferring beliefs and commitments. Schuklenk and Smalling, for example, write:

> Given the intractability of conscience claims, it is not unwarranted to characterise them as essentially arbitrary dislikes.
>
> (2017, 238)

Similarly, Savulescu and Schuklenk question the strength of the beliefs of doctors who conscientiously object to reproductive healthcare interventions or euthanasia. They suggest that

> most people who believe contraception, abortion and euthanasia are wrong don't believe they are evil in the same way as, for example torture and genocide are evil.
>
> (2017, 168)

Conscience, in this respect, might be associated with a series of caprices of agents or, at best, a series of weakly held opinions. Conscience – qua a collection of arbitrary sentiments or opinions – seems far less deserving of respect. One might argue that there is no difference in kind between asking a doctor to disobey their conscience and asking someone who enjoys chocolate ice cream to try a scoop of vanilla ice cream. Both of these requests are concerned with sentiments or preferences even if the former is a more serious request than the latter.

Yet this misrepresents the role of conscience in the psychology of moral agents. Indeed, I take Schuklenk and Smalling's comment to be indicative of one of the most glaring omissions in the literature on conscientious objection, namely a failure to adequately grapple with the moral psychology behind appeals to conscience. As mentioned in the previous chapter, there seems to be a view among some bioethicists that appeals to conscience necessarily involve a commitment to a hopeless form of relativism, whereby people's subjective likes and dislikes are allowed to determine the provision of medical care. I want to argue, however, that conscience claims, insofar as they are sincere and based on a person's deep beliefs, actually track something very morally significant and deserving of respect.

Even those who cautiously support a right to conscientious objection in health-care do not always offer a detailed explanation of the precise moral and existential significance of appeals to conscience. Some theorists appeal to the notion of inner harmony or psychological integrity when attempting to describe the disvalue of acting contrary to conscience. Wicclair, for example, refers to the importance of preserving moral integrity, which he defines as consistency between one's actions and one's core moral convictions (Wicclair 2017, 7–8). Similarly, Childress (1979, 318) associates violations of conscience with a "fundamental loss of integrity, wholeness, and harmony in the self". The question remains, however, as to why a loss of inner harmony or psychological integrity is of disvalue. What is the fundamental problem with acting in a manner that is psychologically discordant?

It is my view that appeals to conscience are actually appeals to the content of one's character, one's conception of morality and, indeed, one's conception of reality. Restrictions on the exercise of conscience, I contend, prevent agents from living in accord with their own considered understanding of the world and the requirements of morality. Related to this, they subvert an agent's pursuit of life projects that give her existence meaning. In what follows, I will offer an account of these moral harms before turning to a consideration of the impact of restrictions of conscience on moral agency.

First, conscience, as we have seen, provides agents with a personal sense of moral obligation. It helps agents to see the requirements of morality in relation to their own self and character. What we are focused on here is not an abstract conception of morality – such as a Kantian deontological framework or a utilitarian framework – which provides only a general and partial account of moral life. Rather, what we are concerned with is an agent's considered understanding of how she ought to act – an understanding of morality formed and sifted through the filter of her own life experiences (Williams 1981). What conscience draws agents' attention to is their own conception of the moral life and their own deep beliefs about their social and professional responsibilities. These beliefs may overlap with a particular universalist conception of moral obligation (be it a Kantian deontological conception of morality, a utilitarian moral theory or some other moral framework). Yet there is no necessary connection between any one particular moral framework and how an individual moral agent understands morality. Ultimately an agent's conception of morality can be as subtly varied as the very variety of human experience itself. Indeed, it is (arguably) through experience and dialogue with others that agents acquire their own rich and deep understanding of morality. What makes an agent's conception of morality *normative* from the perspective of conscience is that it constitutes a fundamental part of her character and her outlook on the world. To reiterate, we are not here focused on some rational imperative or universal law apprehended by the agent. Rather, we are concerned with an agent's sense that she is bound – on pain of violating the content of her own character – to abide by the requirements of morality.

I am here attempting to capture the phenomenology of conscience, rather than making a claim about the nature of morality as such. Two clarifications are in order. First, I am by no means attempting to deny the existence of objective, mind-external moral norms that hold independent of the character and commitments of moral agents. There are certain moral principles that hold always and everywhere. This is compatible with saying that every moral agent has a unique perspective on morality on account of their own unique experience of life and reality. Second, conscience – conceived of as a moral psychological faculty that is worthy of our esteem and respect – necessarily involves some attempt to know reality as it is in itself and not just as it reveals itself to us in our own subjective experience. That is to say, for one's conscience to be deserving of respect, an agent ought to be committed to ensuring that their deeply held beliefs and commitments are compatible with reality and based on evidence from the world. In the words of John Henry Cardinal Newman, "conscience has rights because it has duties" (1964, 383). Conscience has a far weaker claim on respect when it is not grounded in a sincere desire to know reality and to grasp the content of objective morality. One should be open to dialogue and evidence that supports or disproves one's existing commitments.

These caveats notwithstanding, I think that critics like Schuklenk and Smalling are mistaken in the way they characterise the content of conscientious objections, namely as a collection of arbitrary likes and dislikes. Quite on the contrary, for a belief or commitment to form part of an agent's character, it must be something that she has reflectively endorsed and held for some period of time. It must be something that is sincerely felt and that shapes the agent's very outlook on life. Furthermore, it must be underpinned by a genuine desire to know reality and to apprehend the moral order of the universe. Nothing is further from a whim than beliefs and commitments that form the foundation of character.

Here we arrive at a bedrock insight concerning the moral harm of violating conscience. Violations of conscience are not just concerned with the moral distress that an agent experiences when she feels that she has done something seriously wrong. The moral psychological reality is more profound than this. Violations of conscience are concerned with the weakened sense or total loss of self and character that an agent experiences when they transgress their deepest (moral) commitments. Bernard Williams (1981, 13) offers an insightful discussion of this matter, describing an agent's basic commitments or "ground projects" as "the motive force which propels him into the future, and gives him a reason for living". Williams writes:

> [It need not be the case] that if [an agent's ground project] were frustrated or in any of various ways he lost it, he would have to commit suicide, nor does he have to think that . . . but he may feel in those circumstances that he might as well have died . . . in general a man does not have one separable project

which plays this ground role: rather, there is a nexus of projects, related to his conditions of life, and it would be the loss of all or most of them that would remove meaning.

(ibid.)

My claim is that violations of conscience may, in their most serious form, lead to a fundamental loss of meaning and purpose. When an agent not only violates some moral stricture or other but actually abandons their very conception of morality or what makes life worthwhile, they are liable to experience a total loss of purpose and meaning. The impact of a violation of conscience would be worse where an agent violates not just one commitment but the very nexus of commitments that makes their life worthwhile.

Once again, we should remember that the boundary between an agent's moral and non-moral commitments is vague and conceptually problematic (cf. Williams 1981, 14–19). We should be careful about reducing conscience to a series of discrete moral concerns. The norms that form the object of conscience can be as diverse as an agent's own familial, social and professional commitments. The contours of conscience will differ depending on whether we are dealing with a farm owner, a politician, a university lecturer or an intensive care specialist. As Velleman has insightfully observed, conscience has a "diverse portfolio" and is concerned with "volitional necessities [or] obligations of faithfulness to oneself" (2009, 109). The volitional necessities may in some cases be concerned with moral obligation (in the philosopher's sense of the word), yet at other times they will be experienced as non-moral obligations, though obligations nonetheless.

The basic point still stands, however, that conscience is concerned with those actions that are, from the perspective of an agent, "unthinkable". That is to say, conscience is concerned with those actions that an agent "cannot find anything in his self-conception to make it intelligible as something that he would do" (Velleman 2009, 108). To seriously violate conscience is, in a very meaningful sense of the word, to do violence to one's self.

It is appropriate here to deal with a very obvious and pertinent objection. This is, namely, the fact that different moral agents do not seem to experience the effects of conscience in the same way. There is a very real sense in which one reasonable moral agent may find absolutely nothing morally objectionable about an action that another reasonable moral agent sees as being "unthinkable". In what way might my framework accommodate this phenomenon?

I think there are different ways in which we can interpret this objection. First, it may be that one moral agent's considered view of morality coincides with the contents of a conventional moral framework of society or their profession, and so she finds nothing objectionable in what society or their professional role requires her to do. She feels no qualms in abiding by relevant social norms or professional standards. Another moral agent, however, may have arrived at a very different considered view of morality, and, as such, this may come into direct conflict with social convention or the ethical standards of the profession to which they belong. Consider, for example, two doctors, one who believes that access to emergency contraception is a basic human right and another who sees emergency contraception a grave moral evil. There is no contradiction in saying that both agents would be acting reasonably in this situation – even if one were to dispense contraceptives while the other would refrain from doing so.

However, it may also be the case that we are dealing with moral agents who have no moral compass at all. That is to say, there are some situations where a moral agent lacks deep commitments or any sense of integrity. We might, for example, consider the example of a sociopathic, lying businessman who routinely manipulates and deceives his colleagues and clients for his own professional gain. In this case, I would not say that the businessman is tracking some deep aspect of his identity by acting in a manifestly immoral manner. Indeed, the fact that he feels no qualms in deceiving others is evidence of the absence of both conscience *and* deep, character-defining commitments. As Hannah Arendt (1971, 418) writes:

> [O]nly good people are ever bothered by a bad conscience whereas it is a very rare phenomenon among real criminals. A good conscience does not exist except as the absence of a bad one.

"Real criminals", to borrow Arendt's phrase, lack the requisite moral character for conscience to come into play in their moral psychology. They are morally bankrupt individuals and, indeed, only have a moral identity to the extent that they are defined by their morally corrupt actions. Indeed, psychopaths may be another category of person who lack even a bad conscience.

This should suffice for a discussion of the loss of basic meaning and purpose that accompanies a grave violation of conscience. Finally, I would like to discuss the impact of violations of conscience on an agent's capacity for moral agency. It is important to reflect on the criteria according to which we ascribe moral agency to an individual. I would like to focus on two related aspects of agency in particular. First, I would like to focus on the notion that moral agency presupposes a discretionary space in which a moral agent can make moral decisions in an unconstrained way. Second, I would like to focus on the idea that moral agency involves responsibility, whereby one assents to relevant desires and freely wills a particular course of action. Both of these elements of agency are under threat where an external authority seeks to suppress the exercise of conscience.

First, we should recognise that moral agency requires discretionary space in which an agent is free to make their own moral decisions. It may sound like a truism to say that one requires freedom to make free decisions; yet there seems to be widespread confusion about this in the context of social and professional ethics. Some commentators, for example, believe that it is acceptable to enforce professional standards such that a health professional has no option of dissenting from mainstream practice (cf. Stahl and Emanuel 2017). Without the "discretionary space" to choose between different options, however, a moral agent's "choice" of a particular action can only be said to be free in a highly qualified way (cf. Sulmasy 2017). It matters if the moral agent could have chosen otherwise.

If someone's actions were constrained such that she only really had one viable option from which to choose, then she can hardly be said to exercise moral agency in choosing this option. Rather, she would say that her agency has been diminished or distinguished by the constraints that have been imposed on her.

Second, even if we reject the claim that agency requires that an agent has an ability to do otherwise, a moral agent's capacity for agency is, at the very least, conditional on her reflective endorsement of the reasons and desires that motivate her actions. That is to say, for an agent to exercise moral agency, she must reflectively endorse the reasons and desires that lead her to act in particular ways. The agent must have pro-attitudes towards the reasons and desires in question and must desire at a second-order level that the first-order reasons and desires that motivate them actually form part of their will. A failure to do this means that the agent remains "wanton" or indifferent towards the reasons that drive their actions (cf. Frankfurt 1971). This is hardly an example of rational and reflective moral agency.

The trouble with the suppression of conscience, however, is that it involves agents acting on the basis of coercion or compulsion rather than reflectively endorsed desires. If we force people to behave in particular ways, we are not allowing them to act based on reasons and desires that they have reflectively endorsed. Rather, we are leading them to act on the basis of duress, and there is a very real sense in which they are not exercising their agency – at least, not in the fullest sense of the word. For example, if someone commits a crime in the heat of passion, there is a sense in which her responsibility for that crime is diminished. She has not fully reflectively endorsed their course of action and so cannot be said to be acting with the full force of her character. I would argue that something analogous is occurring when social or professional norms are enforced in such a way that individual moral agents have no choice but to conform to these norms. An agent's adherence to such norms is motivated by an external force rather than by a rationally endorsed, interior conviction that one ought to act in accord with these norms.

It is instructive here to return to the idea of integrity and to consider how this might be related to agency. Part of what it means to be a moral agent is to have principles and to act consistently in accord with these principles. MacIntyre (1999, 317) links integrity to maintenance of a fixed identity and suggests that it underpins one's existence as an integrated person. He writes:

> To have integrity is to refuse to be, to have educated oneself so that one is no longer able to be, one kind of person in one social context, while quite another in other contexts. It is to have set inflexible limits to one's adaptability to the roles that one may be called upon to play.

Some theorists may argue that adaptability is a virtue, particularly when one is discharging an important social or professional role. That is to say, it could be argued that it is virtuous to make oneself amenable to the relevant conventions that one encounters in one's social or professional life. I would argue, however, that adaptability is only a virtue when one has manifestly fallen into moral error. In contrast, where one is indeed convinced upon reflection that one has arrived at the correct moral conviction vis-à-vis one's social or professional obligations, it is a virtue rather than a vice to hold to one's beliefs rather than adapting to the demands that have been placed on oneself by one's peers. This is precisely what it means to have integrity. Conscience, for its part, is that aspect of our psychology that leads us to maintain integrity and to persist in our beliefs and commitments when these conflict with prevailing social or professional norms.

Agency follows on from integrity, as agency is about acting in a manner consonant with one's beliefs and commitments. Those beliefs and commitments that are most truly our own are those that have been sifted through reflection and experience and that we have interiorised to form part of our character. We exercise moral agency, in the fullest sense of the word, when we act *wholeheartedly* (Frankfurt 1988). This wholeheartedness in turn requires at least some degree of inflexibility (enough inflexibility for us to maintain some grip on our own personal identity).

Agents who abandon their deeply held beliefs also undermine their capacity for independent moral judgement. Our personal moral ideals are an epistemic standpoint from which we can independently judge the professional norms and standards that are imposed on us. They allow us to "step outside" of our professional role and view the world from our own unique moral point of view, which has been shaped over the course of many years. By setting "inflexible limits" on the kinds of social and professional functions that we are willing to perform, we maintain epistemic and volitional independence from the social and professional communities of which we form a part. To the extent that we lack personal moral ideals, however – or to the extent that we allow these ideals to be eroded – we lose the vantage point from which we can independently critique the norms that characterise our social and professional communities. If the moral content of our character becomes indistinguishable from the moral conventions of these communities – or, perhaps more to the point, if we fail to sift these conventions through the filter of our own capacity for critical reflection – we lose the capacity for impartial and detached judgement that is necessary to externally critique social or professional conventions. If we are endlessly willing to adapt ourselves to any convention that is foisted upon us, we will lose the agential independence necessary to externally critique the communities of practice of which we form a part.

– A problem with the suppression of conscience, then, is that it undermines those features of moral rationality that are prerequisite of agency. Agents are encouraged to suppress and abandon those beliefs that ultimately form the bedrock of their understanding of the world. Rather, they are led to make themselves fully beholden to professional moral standards rather than following their own beliefs about what is right and wrong. These factors combine to undermine an agent's capacity for independent moral judgement, which presumably is a core feature of moral agency. The suppression of conscience, in this sense, greatly diminishes an agent's capacity for considered moral judgement and action independent of the norms internal to social practices.

Conclusion

In this chapter, I have provided an account of the role that conscience plays in moral life. I argued that conscience is a principle of moral awareness in human beings and that it gives agents an awareness of the personal relevance of moral obligation. I then offered an overview of the loss of character and purpose that agents experience when they violate their conscience. I argued that moral agents risk losing their basic orienting ideals if they act in a manner contrary to their deep moral and other normative commitments. Agents who abandon their deeply held beliefs, furthermore, also undermine their capacity for independent moral judgement. Our personal moral ideals are an epistemic standpoint from which we can independently judge the social and professional norms of the communities of practice to which we belong. To the extent that one lacks personal moral ideals, or one allows these ideals to be eroded, one loses the vantage point from which one can independently critique the norms of professional work and social life.

There is much more we could say about conscience and moral psychology, yet it is more important for our purposes to consider more specifically how conscience applies to professional life. In the next chapter, we will discuss in greater detail the role that conscience plays in professional practice and, particularly, healthcare practice. I will argue that we should respect conscientious objectors in medicine because professional discretion is integral to the cultivation of virtue and character; virtue and character, in turn, facilitate the realisation of the goods of medicine. Insofar as we restrict a doctor's right to professional discretion, however, we restrict a doctor's capacity to fulfil their professional role. This has serious, negative implications for both individual practitioners and the medical profession itself.

Notes

1 To be clear, Sulmasy (2008) rejects this view. His own view is much closer to my own.
2 It is apposite to clarify how I am using the term "practical reason". My understanding of this capacity of the mind leans heavily in the direction of Aristotle and Aquinas. Practical reason – in the sense that I am using the term – refers to the capacity of the human mind for reasoning and judgement about human action. It is concerned with how we ought to act and behave, rather than speculative or theoretical matters. Practical reason is responsible for applying the first principles of morality to particular real-world moral situations.
3 The judgements of practical reason, in other words, form part of the content of conscience. If practical reason errs, then conscience will err, too.
4 For an insightful discussion of non-moral forms of guilt and shame, see David Velleman. *How We Get Along*. New York: Cambridge University Press, 2009: 97–100.

References

Anscombe, Elizabeth. *Human Life, Action and Ethics: Essays by G.E.M. Anscombe*. Exeter: Imprint Academia, 2005.

Arendt, Hannah. "Lying in politics: Reflections on the Pentagon Papers". *The New York Review of Books* 18th November 1971 ed.

Audi, Robert, and Murphy, Patrick. "The many faces of integrity". *Business Ethics Quarterly* 16;1 (2006): 3–21.

Benjamin, Martin. "Conscience". In Warren T. Reich (ed.). *Encyclopedia of Bioethics Volume 1* (2nd ed.). Basingstoke: Macmillan, 1995: 469–472.

Blustein, Jeffrey. "Doing what the patient orders: Maintaining integrity in the doctor-patient relationship". *Bioethics* 7;4 (1993): 289–314.

Butler, Joseph. *Fifteen Sermons Preached at the Rolls Chapel.* London: Botham, 1950 [1726].

Childress, James. "Appeals to conscience". *Ethics* 89;4 (1979): 315–335; 328.

Cottingham, John. "Conscience, guilt, and shame". In Roger Crisp (ed.). *The Oxford Handbook of the History of Ethics.* London: Oxford University Press, 2013: 729–743; 733.

Cullity, Garrett. "Moral virtues and responsiveness for reasons". In Stewart Braun and Noell Birondo (eds.). *Virtue's Reasons: New Essays on Virtue, Character, and Reasons.* New York: Routledge, 2017: 11–31.

D'Arcy, Eric. *Conscience and Its Right to Freedom.* New York: Sheed and Ward, 1961.

Fernandez Lynch, Holly. *Conflicts of Conscience in Health Care: An Institutional Compromise.* MIT Press, 2008.

Frankfurt, Harry. "Alternate possibilities and moral responsibility". *Journal of Philosophy* 66 (1969): 829–839.

Frankfurt, Harry. "Freedom of the will and the concept of a person". *Journal of Philosophy* 68 (1971): 5–20.

Frankfurt, Harry. *The Importance of What We Care About.* New York: Cambridge University Press, 1988.

Fuss, Peter. "Conscience". *Ethics* 74;2 (1964): 111–120.

Hanna, Deborah. "The lived experience of moral distress: Nurses who assisted with elective abortions". *Research Theory and Nursing Practice* 19;1 (2005): 95–124.

Hawthorne, Nathaniel. *The Scarlet Letter.* London: Oxford University Press, 2007.

Hill, Thomas. "Four conceptions of conscience". *Nous* 40 (1998): 13–52.

Hoffmann, Tobias. "Conscience and synderesis". In Brian Davies (ed.). *The Oxford Handbook of Aquinas.* London: Oxford University Press, 2012: 255–262.

Hume, David. *A Treatise of Human Nature.* London: Oxford Clarendon Press, 1975.

Kant, Immanuel. *The Metaphysics of Morals.* Mary Gregor (trans.). Cambridge: Cambridge University Press, 2017.

Keiran, Matthew. "Art and morality". In Jerrold Levison (ed.). *The Oxford Handbook of Aesthetics.* London: Oxford University Press, 2003: 451–470.

Kodelja, Zdenko. "The voice of conscience in Rousseau's Emile". *Ethics and Education* 10;2 (2015): 198–208.

Langston, Douglas. *Conscience and Other Virtues: From Bonaventure to MacIntyre.* State College: Penn State University Press, 2001.

Lyons, William. "Conscience: An essay in moral psychology". *Philosophy* 84;4 (2009): 477–494.

MacIntyre, Alistair. "Social structures and their threats to moral agency". *Philosophy* 74;3 (1999): 311–329.

McFall, Lynn. "Integrity". *Ethics* 98;1 (1987): 5–20.

McLeod, Carolyn. *Conscience in Reproductive Health Care: Prioritising Patient Interests.* New York: Oxford University Press, 2020.

Moral Injury Project. "What is moral injury". Syracuse: Syracuse University, 2014. Available from https://moralinjuryproject.syr.edu/about-moral-injury/.

Newman, John Henry. "Letter to the Duke of Norfolk". In Francis X. Connolly (ed.). *A Newman Reader*. Garden City, NY: Doubleday, 1964: 383.

Ojakangas, Mika. *The Voice of Conscience: A Political Genealogy of Western Ethical Experience*. London: Bloomsbury, 2013.

O'Shea, Tom. "Modern moral conscience". *International Journal of Philosophical Studies* 26;4 (2018): 582–600.

Ramsay, Hayden. *Beyond Virtue: Integrity and Morality*. London: MacMillan, 1997.

Rousseau, Jean Jacques. *Emile: Or on Education*. Barbara Foxley (trans.). London & Toronto: J.M. Dent and Sons; New York: E.P. Dutton, 1921 [1762].

Saad, Toni C. Conscientious objection and clinical judgement: The right to refuse to harm. *The New Bioethics* 25;3 (2019): 248–261.

Savulescu, Julian, and Schuklenk, Udo. "Doctors have no right to refuse medical assistance in dying, abortion or contraception". *Bioethics* 31;3 (2017): 162–170.

Schiller, Fredrich. "On grace and dignity". Jane V. Curran (trans.). In Jane V. Curran and Christophe Fricker (eds.). *Schiller's "On Grace and Dignity' in Its Cultural Context: Essays and a New Translation*. Rochester, NY: Camden House, 2005: 123–170.

Schinkel, Anders. *Conscience and Conscientious Objections*. Amsterdam: Vrije Universiteit, 2007.

Schinkel, Anders. *Conscience and Conscientious Objections*. Amsterdam: Amsterdam University Press, 2007.

Schuklenk, Udo, and Smalling, Ricardo. "Why medical professionals have no moral claim to conscientious objection accommodation in liberal democracies". *Journal of Medical Ethics* 43 (2017): 234–240; 238.

Shaftesbury, Anthony A.C. *Characteristics of Men, Manners, Opinions and Times*. London: Cambridge University Press, 1999.

Stahl, Ronit, and Emanuel, Ezekiel. "Physicians not conscripts; conscientious objection in healthcare". *The New England Journal of Medicine* 376;14 (2017): 1380–1385.

Stoker, Hendrik. *Conscience: Phenomena and Theories*. Phillip E. Blosser (trans.). South Bend: University of Notre Dame Press, 2018.

Strohm, Paul. *Conscience: A Very Short Introduction*. London: Oxford University Press, 2011.

Sulmasy, Daniel. "What is conscience and why is respect for it so important". *Theoretical Medicine and Bioethics* 29 (2008): 135–149; 138.

Sulmasy, Daniel. "Tolerance, professional judgement, and the discretionary space of the physician". *Cambridge Quarterly of Healthcare Ethics* 21;6 (2017): 18–31.

Velleman, David. *How We Get Along*. New York: Cambridge University Press, 2009.

Wicclair, Mark. *Conscientious Objection in Health Care: An Ethical Analysis*. New York: Cambridge University Press, 2011.

Wicclair, Mark. "Conscientious objection in healthcare and moral integrity". *Cambridge Quarterly of Healthcare Ethics* 26;1 (2017): 7–17.

Williams, Bernard. "Persons, character, and morality". In Williams, Bernard (ed.). *Moral Luck: Philosophical Papers 1973–80*. Cambridge: Cambridge University Press, 1981: 1–19.

Wood, Allen. *Kantian Ethics*. New York: Cambridge University Press, 2008.

4   A theory of conscience – part II

Virtue, character and conscientious objection in medical practice

Introduction

In the previous chapter I offered a detailed account of the role of conscience in moral life. This chapter considers how a virtue and character-based model of medicine can inform our understanding of the ethics of conscientious objection in healthcare practice. I argue that the exercise of conscience is integral to the practice of medicine and, by implication, that we ought to permit conscientious objection. Freedom of conscience is necessary if physicians are to cultivate the virtues constitutive of excellence in medicine. It is through free action and the exercise of one's capacity for independent clinical judgement that doctors acquire the virtues constitutive of excellence in medical practice (Pellegrino and Thomasma 1993). In light of this, healthcare professionals should be given significant professional freedom to choose how they will practise medicine and to determine how they will pursue the goods that are the end (telos) of medical practice.

To be clear, the central argument of this chapter is concerned with the value of cultivating conscience in medical practice. Medicine has both technical and moral dimensions, and doctors must learn to exercise their capacity for technical and moral judgement. This will often involve a process of consultation with one's peers. Doctors should give due consideration to the recommendations that are made by other clinicians, particularly where those clinicians have privileged epistemic access to relevant medical theory and clinical facts. Yet we must also acknowledge the important role that personal reflection and the exercise of one's independent capacity for clinical judgement play in the cultivation of professional virtues.[1] Virtues are not acquired in a passive fashion but require rational deliberation and volition on the part of an agent. It is with this in mind that I offer a character and virtue-based account of medicine and discuss the importance of "discretionary space" for medical practitioners (Sulmasy 2017).

Section 1 of this chapter outlines a goal directed model of medicine that emphasises the importance of the cultivation of character and virtue. I introduce the notion of a physician's discretionary space and argue that the protection of this discretionary space is necessary if physicians are to acquire the virtues constitutive of excellence in medicine. In Section 2, I consider how conscientious objection forms part of a physician's discretionary space. I argue that respect for physician

DOI: 10.4324/9781003247623-4

discretion involves a presumption in favour of permitting individual conscientious objection. In Section 3 I offer an account of what constitutes reasonable disagreement about the nature of medicine.

1. A virtue- and character-based conception of medical practice

In this section I will explore a conception of medical practice that focuses on virtue, character and moral agency and that uses these concepts as a lens through which to understand medical professionalism. The provider of services model of medicine (PSM) offers an implausible account of medicine and sets up a conflict between individual medical professionals and the norms of the medical profession. I will argue that virtue, character and moral agency are essential aspects of medical professionalism. What's more, one cannot adequately understand the phenomenon of conscientious objection without coming to terms with the prior notions of professional discretion and the cultivation of virtue in clinical practice. This discussion, therefore, will explore the nature of medical practice and will consider why the cultivation of professional virtue is essential to good medical practice.

The provider of services model of medicine

The PSM (Curlin and Tollefsen 2019, 2021) holds that medicine has a transactional nature and is essentially about the delivery of a service, namely healthcare. According to this view, medicine is analogous to any other form of service provision within our society, such as driving a cab or providing cleaning services. Consumer preferences should determine the kinds of services that are provided and the manner in which they are provided. The role of clinicians is to provide medical services requested by patients; a doctor's ethical duties are based around the fulfilment of this role.

A corollary of this is that doctors should not allow their personal views to affect the way in which they interact with patients. Patients should have access to all safe and legal medical services, and a doctor's privately held moral or religious beliefs should not be allowed to impact on the availability of medical procedures. As Stahl and Emanuel write, physicians may believe what they will "in their private lives . . . but in their role as health care professionals, they must provide the appropriate interventions as specified by the medical profession" (2017, 1383). The medical profession, for its part, should seek to ensure that healthcare services are readily available for all consumers. The profession should seek to reduce barriers to patient access, be these financial or locational barriers or barriers arising from a physician's own personal moral reservations about safe and legal medical procedures. Patients should be able to access healthcare services in a manner that is timely and convenient.

As we observed in Chapter 2, PSM fosters a problematic ethic of compliance in medicine rather than focusing on the virtue and character of clinicians. It hollows out traditional models of medical professionalism and replaces them with a government and market-focused account of medical practice. Most relevant to our purposes, the PSM sets up a conflict between the exercise of conscience and the fundamental norms of the profession. The norms of professional associations are given a kind of absolute importance while conscience is consigned to the realm of one's private beliefs. This creates a situation in which the exercise of conscience is seen as being irrelevant to good clinical judgement. Indeed, the moral views of individual practitioners are portrayed as suspicious and potentially harmful to the well-being of patients. This is a problematic situation in a profession which is characterised by a multiplicity of ethically complex situations and that requires that its practitioners foster a capacity for sound ethical judgement.

A goal-directed model of medicine

The model of medicine I would like to defend departs from the PSM insofar as it conceives of medicine as a practice that is directed towards certain goods – in particular, the goods of health and healing – and argues that the exercise of conscience is essential to discerning how these goods apply in particular situations. Rather than consigning conscience to the realm of one's private beliefs, a goal-directed model of medicine acknowledges the moral character of the medical endeavour and recognises conscience as an indispensable feature of the moral psychology of virtuous medical practitioners. The virtuous practitioner is one who is skilled in discerning and pursuing the medical and human good in the multiplicity of circumstances that characterise contemporary medical practice. A well-cultivated conscience gives practitioners a special sensitivity for discerning the goods of health and healing by leading them to take account of relevant clinical and moral considerations, relevant law and professional guidelines, the wishes and preferences of patients, and one's own acquired wisdom as an experienced medical practitioner.

In saying that medicine is directed to the goods of health and healing, I mean not only that doctors ought to act in the service of these goods but also that we cannot understand medicine without having these goods in view. Doctors are in the business of saving lives and treating illness and injury; we could not make sense of the role of doctors without a focus on their therapeutic acts. Medicine is unintelligible if we fail to take into account its basic orientation towards life and health. My claim, then, is not just a descriptive claim about what doctors do. It is also a metaphysical claim about the nature of medicine as a social practice and the fact that it is defined by these goods. Medicine is *teleological*, insofar as it is a practice that is defined by the goods at which it aims. I here have in mind MacIntyre's conception of practice as a "coherent and complex form of socially established cooperative human activity" with its own internal goods and standards of excellence (MacIntyre 1997, 187). Medicine is a coordinated human activity which is directed towards the goods of health and healing, and it has its own virtues which arise from these goods (Figure 4.1).

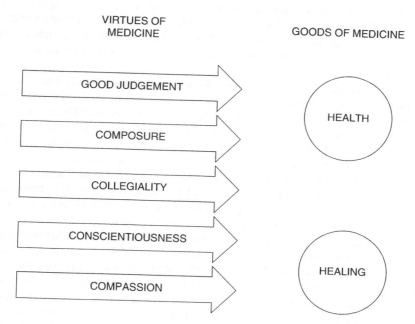

VIRTUES OF
MEDICINE

GOODS OF MEDICINE

GOOD JUDGEMENT

COMPOSURE

COLLEGIALITY

CONSCIENTIOUSNESS

COMPASSION

HEALTH

HEALING

Figure 4.1 The goods and virtues of medicine

In contrast to PSM, this model rejects the idea that medicine is solely concerned with service-provision, respect for patient rights and welfare, and/or the promotion of patient preferences. This is not to say that we should ignore patient rights and welfare; these are indeed important considerations that should inform the decision-making of healthcare practitioners. This model, however, conceives of patient rights and welfare *within the context of the medical good*. The scope and limits of patient rights and welfare are determined by the scope and limits of what one takes to be constitutive of health and healing (Sulmasy 2002). It would not make sense for a doctor to honour a patient's request for a service that was manifestly contrary to the goods of health and healing. A patient with xenomelia might, for example, ask a clinician for assistance in amputating a perfectly healthy limb.[2] It would be contrary to the goals of medicine, however, for the doctor to assist the patient in doing this, notwithstanding the patient's intense desires to cut off a healthy limb.

Not everyone would agree with the idea that doctors should not perform certain interventions that are contrary to the traditional goods of medicine. There is ongoing debate about whether medicine is in fact a social practice with its own ethical code (sometimes described as the internal morality of medicine) or whether medicine is in fact governed by an external ethical framework such as an ethic of preference satisfaction and respect for autonomy or some more fundamental ethical system based on a conception of human flourishing. Depending on one's view on this issue, one may have different attitudes towards the normative status of controversial medical procedures such as limb amputations for patients with xenomelia. I will not canvas this debate, however, as it would distract us from the central focus of this chapter.

Suffice to say that the *core of medicine* is characterised by a focus on health and healing. A useful framework that provides justification for this claim is Miller, Brody and Cheng's tripartite account of the normative status of different medical interventions and practices (2001). Miller, Brody and Cheng suggest that we can distinguish medical interventions that (i) lie at the core of medicine from (ii) medical interventions that are "borderline" or "peripheral" and (iii)other interventions that uncontroversially violate the goals of medical practice. Medical interventions that uncontroversially promote the goals of medicine would include clinically indicated interventions like treating bacterial infections with antibiotics or using clot-busting medication to treat an ischemic stroke. No one would dispute that these sorts of interventions fall within the purview of medicine. According to the authors, "borderline" or "peripheral" medical interventions are those "which belong within the legitimate domain of medicine but are not clearly supported by the goals of medicine and seem to conflict to some extent with one or more of the internal duties" (2000, 356). Examples that they provide are the provision of contraceptives or the performance of sterilisation operations. These interventions may be controversial in some contexts or for some practitioners as they disrupt sexual function. Most professional associations would, nevertheless, consider them part of the full suite of services that medicine should provide to society. Examples of practices that uncontroversially violate the goals of medicine are physician participation in capital punishment and the provision of anabolic steroids to athletes for the purposes of performance enhancement (Miller, Brody and Cheng 2000, 356). It is very difficult for someone to defend these practices as having a place in medicine.[3]

This should suffice for a discussion of the teleological model of medical practice, namely a model focused on the goods of health and healing. In sum, our understanding of medicine ought to have as its reference the goods of health and healing, at least insofar as we are concerned with the "core of legitimate medical practice" (Miller, Brody and Cheng 2000, 356).[4] This is the closest we can get to a definition of the basic aims of medicine, and it stands to reason that our conception of medical professionalism should have as its focus these medical goods.[5]

Virtue in medical practice

Proponents of a goal-directed model of medicine place significant emphasis on the cultivation of virtue and character in medical practitioners (Pellegrino and Thomasma 1993, 1996). This is in contrast to other medico-ethical frameworks, which tend to focus on duties to the exclusion of virtues. By virtues, I have in mind habits of excellence that allow practitioners to realise the goods of medicine. The virtues of medicine are the habits that clinicians must have if they are to achieve excellence in their professional role. We might, for example, think of the virtues of reliability, collegiality, composure, personality, good judgement, transparency and so forth. For a clinician to be considered not only competent but a model of professional excellence, they must exhibit at least some if not all of these virtues. We should also consider those virtues that are associated more explicitly with the exercise of conscience, namely integrity, fidelity to one's professional calling and habits of moral reflection. For a clinician to be committed to their profession and to have a habit of learning from their mistakes, they must cultivate the moral awareness and fidelity that is attended upon the exercise of conscience.

Building on this notion of virtue, one could say that the medical profession has an interest in training virtuous medical practitioners – practitioners who have a strong capacity for moral discernment, reflection and reasoned decision-making and who have a strong sense of vocation in the way that they approach their work. We want doctors to embody the sorts of virtues that we take to be constitutive of good medical practice, and so we should look at ways in which we can encourage doctors and make space for them to acquire these virtues that we take to be constitutive of good medical care (Weinstock 2014, 11–12). Medical educators and associations should identify educational methods and formative initiatives that promote rather than hinder practitioners' cultivation of virtue (Hawking, Curlin and Yoon 2017).

We should, in sum, seek to create a culture in which physicians are led to acquire the professional character traits that are integral to good medical practice. Indeed, Beauchamp and Childress, who are best known as pioneers of a principlist approach to bioethics, argued that medical practitioners should cultivate virtues such as "compassion, discernment, trustworthiness, integrity, and conscientiousness" (Garcia 2020). Virtue ethics should not be seen as a niche interest of a small minority of bioethicists interested in Aristotle or Christian ethics.

The formation of virtuous medical practitioners

It is important, here, to consider how the moral and professional formation of doctors occurs. The end point of practitioner education is that clinicians acquire the professional virtues necessary to realise the goods that are at the centre of medicine. Virtues allow doctors to identify the goods of medicine in particular situations and to pursue these goods in an excellent manner. The cultivation of virtue and the cultivation of character, furthermore, are inextricably linked. One dimension of the cultivation of virtue is the interiorisation of moral beliefs and commitments. When a moral agent interiorises beliefs and commitments these beliefs and commitments come to form the horizons of intelligible moral action for the agent and provide the agent with moral motivation and moral guidance. These interiorised beliefs and commitments are surely a constitutive feature of character (understood as a stable set of dispositions that inform motivation and guide conduct).

Building on this account of virtue and character, we can say that medical professionalism requires the interiorisation of the values of medicine (AMA 2010).

Healthcare professionals must interiorise a conception of what constitutes good medical practice and must – through their own experience as well as through guidance from peers – cultivate a capacity for discerning the medical good in particular circumstances. They must constitute their own moral and technical rationality such that they can correctly identify how the medical good ought to be realised in particular situations in clinical practice. This is an essential part of one's formation as a virtuous medical practitioner.

Part of this process of professional formation involves acquiring a knowledge of relevant guidelines and learning from one's peers. Medicine, after all, is a community of inquiry and practice, and one comes to be part of this community through a process of epistemic and normative initiation (Cruess, Cruess and Steinert 2018; Symons 2019). One learns from the experience and testimony of others, and one interiorises the moral and technical advice that has been passed on to one by other more experienced clinicians (Arthur *et al.* 2015, 30). Professional standards and norms, furthermore, have a very important place in the practice of medicine. They provide an outline of the contours of medicine as a practice and give doctors clear ethical guidance about acceptable practice in medicine. It is hard to overstate the role that this plays in the professional formation of new clinicians. Professional standards and norms also provide reassurance to patients, healthcare administrations and politicians that medicine is not being practised in a disorganised and unprincipled fashion – which is important if medicine is to retain society's trust.

For these reasons, professional detachment and epistemic humility form an important part of a medical practitioner's professional formation. By epistemic humility, I have in mind a respect for the clinical judgement of one's peers. We might, for example, think of a junior doctor in an intensive care unit who believes that continued life support for an apparently brain-dead patient may potentially be appropriate but who defers to a more senior clinician who says that life support should be discontinued. Respect for professional standards and the opinion of one's peers are an essential feature of collegiality and prudent decision-making in medicine. Healthcare professionals should have a healthy sense of their own limitations and their need to learn from the perspective of their peers, particularly more experienced peers (Wilkinson 2017). Individual practitioners should, furthermore, practise within the bounds of what can reasonably be construed as medical practice.[6] No single medical practitioner should take themselves to be the sole authority on what constitutes good medical care, even if they choose to follow their conscience in some situations where they disagree with the prevailing understanding of the medical good. At the very least, practitioners should give significant epistemic weight to the opinions of other members of the medical community. We should not underestimate, therefore, the importance of epistemic humility in medical practice.

It would, however, be naive to limit our understanding of professional formation in medicine to a passive reception of wisdom via one's peers and the guidance of professional associations. One's own moral reflection and experience practising as a doctor is also crucial to the acquisition of virtue. Virtue cannot just be taught – it must be also acquired through activity. Virtues are habits and so become part of the psychology and identity of agents through free and repeated action (cf. Aristotle's *Ethics* 1103a20–1). In the case of medicine, doctors must learn to exercise their capacity for technical and moral judgement to determine what the medical good is in a particular situation. This will often involve a process of consultation with one's peers, particularly where one's peers have privileged epistemic access to relevant medical theory and clinical facts. Yet we must also acknowledge the indispensable role of personal reflection and the exercise of one's independent capacity for clinical judgement in the cultivation of professional virtues. Consider, for example, if one found oneself as a junior clinician involved in the infamous Tuskegee Syphilis Experiment of the 1930s to 1970s.[7] It would be the height of negligence if one were to passively rely on the morally bankrupt judgements of seniors or peers or if one were to ignore one's own moral intuitions about the ethics of withholding medical treatment for syphilis from study participants. Rather, one ought to exercise one's own capacity for moral judgement in such a situation and blow the whistle on what is a manifestly unethical trial.

Virtues are not acquired in a passive fashion but instead require rational deliberation and volition on the part of an agent. In the case of medicine, a doctor must desire to acquire virtue and cultivate their capacity for clinical judgement so that they can learn to effectively manage the multifarious clinical situations that arise in the course of the practice of medicine.[8] This process requires that we give doctors *space* to exercise their capacity for judgement. The impulse driving much of the literature on conscientious objection is the idea that the medical profession must reliably deliver healthcare services to consumers and that we should seek to regulate medical practice such that the reliable delivery of services is guaranteed (Charo 2005; Savulescu 2006; Minerva 2015). Yet an attempt to micromanage and restrict the decision-making of medical practitioners ignores the importance of giving clinicians space to cultivate and sustain their capacities for clinical and moral judgement. Rather than attempting to prescribe norms for every single clinical situation a doctor may encounter, we should look to respect clinicians' legitimate exercise of their technical and moral rationality. With this in mind, we will now turn to the topic of a *physician's discretionary space*.

The physician's discretionary space

In this section I will offer an overview of the notion of a physician's discretionary space and will consider how it is related to the cultivation of character and virtue in medicine. Much could be said about the utility of professional dissensus for moral and technical progress in medicine. This itself is an argument for giving physicians broad latitude to practise in accord with their own understanding of medical practice. Yet I will not base my defence of discretionary freedoms on the value of disagreement and dissensus in prompting progress in the medical profession. I will instead focus on the importance of professional discretion in the cultivation of virtue and character.

Physicians must have at least some degree of professional freedom if they are to cultivate the virtues constitutive of medical practice. With this in mind, we should seek to maintain and protect a *physician's discretionary space*. By this, I am referring to a space for individual technical and moral discernment for clinicians whereby they are allowed to determine whether a particular intervention or practice would be conducive to the goods of health and health-related well-being or whether in fact the intervention would be harmful to a patient. Clinicians should, as a rule, be allowed to form their own judgement about the value or disvalue of particular treatments and whether these treatments are suitable for particular patients. They should be given latitude to practise in accord with their own considered understanding of what constitutes good medicine (Saad 2019).

This emphasis on individual discretion, while it refers to individual moral agents, should not be reduced to a personal project of moral development. It is vitally important to the pursuit of excellence in medicine. Sulmasy (2017) writes:

> Society has an interest in promoting good medicine, and, therefore, society has an interest in granting physicians the wide discretionary space that is required to make medical practice excellent. All algorithms are ultimately only guidelines. Medicine may be scientifically informed, but medical practice is ultimately an art and not a science.
>
> (p. 24)

There is no conceivable way in which medical associations or health authorities could micromanage medical practice such that the need for professional discretion was rendered null and void. Medicine is concrete, variable and context-dependent, and patients are complex individuals rather than homogenous cases. This makes considered individual practitioner judgement a vital component of good medicine.

To be clear, a physician's discretionary space is most important because of the connection it bears to virtue, character and the acquisition of a professional identity. Without space to exercise their agency, physicians will never acquire the character and virtue that are required for the realisation of the goods internal to the medical profession. Indeed, one cannot have virtue without agency, and all the more so in medicine where expertise is clearly acquired through one's experience making decisions in a clinical context. The professional wisdom that distinguishes an excellent clinician from an average one is often based on "what they don't teach in med school" – things as simple and human as "hand-holding and winning trust" (Makary 2014). Without the space to exercise their capacities for moral and technical discernment and action, however, physicians will fail to develop the traits necessary for excellence in medical practice. Professional discretion is necessary for doctors to be able to interiorise the values of care and conscientiousness that we take to be central to the medical profession.

The previous chapter argued that we should give moral agents broad scope in which to exercise their conscience, as conscience monitors the extent to which an agent is being faithful to her own conception of morality and other basic commitments. What we did not discuss, however, is the process whereby one acquires character-defining commitments. I noted in passing that it is through experience and dialogue with one's peers that one comes to acquire their own understanding of morality. I did not, however, discuss the importance of communities of practice in shaping one's commitments and identity, nor did I explore how one comes to form part of a community of practice. It is apposite to consider this matter now, if only briefly.

Character is formed (at least in part) through the acquisition of central life commitments that provide a sense of meaning and purpose to one's life. These central commitments are what define the moral identity of agents and shape their view of the world. In the case of doctors, it is important that they have a strong sense of professional belonging such that their profession becomes a central life commitment and to some extent informs their outlook on their own social and professional lives. Indeed, I would argue that a virtuous clinician is someone who has a vocational sense of their own professional role – not necessarily in the sense that they feel a *calling* to medicine but simply in the sense that they feel that their professional occupation is part of their identity and that they form part of a community of inquiry and practice. With this in view, there is a sense in which it would be "out of character" for a doctor to wilfully act in a manner contrary to the goals of medical practice. Professional ethics, for the virtuous physician, is not just about what external guidelines flag as permissible or non-permissible actions. Professional ethics is about who one is at the level of character and the horizon of moral actions that one can intentionally engage in without contravening the very essence of one's professional identity. To return to our earlier discussion we should remember that medicine is a goal-directed practice and that concepts such as virtue and patient welfare are defined in reference to the goals of medicine, namely goods like health and healing. Professional ethics is about making these goods the object of one's professional practice allowing them to inform one's moral and technical rationality.

Crucially, the way in which doctors acquire a sense of professional identity – conceived of as a feature of their own character and self – is through a process of inculturation in the medical profession. Through training, experience, erudition, dialogue with peers and reflection, doctors come to form part of the community of practice that is medicine (Cruess, Cruess and Steinert 2018; Symons 2019). This is not just a one-way process of instruction in which individual clinicians are just passive participants. Rather, clinicians must actively engage with and interiorise the technical and moral rationality that characterises medicine. This requires reflection and a considered and sustained choice on the part of the practitioner, in addition to a willingness of the profession to receive them. The individual moral agent must make a conscious and ongoing commitment to becoming a member of the medical profession and seeking to realise the goods of the profession with distinction. This is precisely why the idea of *profession* in medicine is important. Without some sort of fundamental personal commitment at the heart of medical practice – that is, the commitments to patients and to society that a doctor *professes to make* – it would be difficult to see how doctors could develop the sense of professional identity, commitment and purpose that we take to be constitutive of virtue in medicine. I am here relying upon Pellegrino and Thomasma's account

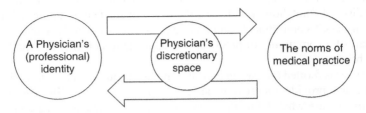

Figure 4.2 Professional identity, physician discretion and professional norms

of a profession as involving "a public promise – a 'profession' – that the new physician understands the gravity of his or her calling, promises to be competent, and promises to use that competence in the interests of the sick" (1993, 36). Admittedly, not all medical schools require their graduates to take an oath or make a public profession, but it is plausible to suggest that some sort of public commitment is implied in one's joining of the medical profession (Figure 4.2).[9]

A corollary of this is that we should safeguard the discretionary space of a physician. The discretionary space of a physician is the moral domain in which a physician's identity is constituted and where medical ethics goes from being a mere exercise in compliance to constituting the very fabric of one's character. Insofar as we want clinicians to have a deep commitment to fulfilling their professional role and to conscientiously carry out their professional duties, we should protect a physician's discretionary space. With this in mind, we will now consider the relationship between a physician's discretionary space and the practice of conscientious objection in healthcare.

2. Physician discretion and conscientious objection

It is apposite to consider the implications of our discussion so far for the practice of conscientious objection. Specifically, we should consider how a physician's discretionary space relates to conscientious objection. In this section, I will argue that the practice of conscientious objection is, in many if not most instances, underpinned by disagreements about the goods of medicine and how best to realise these goods in clinical practice. I will argue that these disagreements fall within the discretionary space of a physician and that dissenting clinicians should be respected for this reason. I will also respond to a series of objections that critics of conscientious objection have made of practitioners who seek to act in accord with their deeply held moral convictions.

First, conscientious objections are in many, if not most cases, characterised by a physician's dissenting view of the nature of the goods of medicine. That is to say, conscientious objection is not (or, at least, not always) discontinuous with ordinary clinical disagreements about how a treating team should provide care to a patient. What we are dealing with in the case of many conscientious objections is an exercise of a physician's moral and technical judgement concerning how the medical good ought to be realised in a particular situation. This sort of disagreement is not about one's religious or personal values. The question is, rather, about how we should think about the goods of medicine in particular situations and how these goods would be best realised. Kim and Ferguson (2021) call these Nature of Medicine Conscientious Objections (NoMCOs).

Herein lies a very important insight: conscientious objectors ought not to be glibly accused of imposing their personal values on their patients. Rather, in many cases the issue is a disagreement about the goods at the centre of medical practice and how we ought to go about realising these goods. This kind of conscientious objector thinks that a particular medical practice in general or in some particular subset of situations is not conducive to health and health-related well-being. Polemical rhetoric about physician paternalism and the imposition of values, therefore, should be treated with caution. When Schuklenk and Smalling characterise conscientious objection as an expression of doctors' vague "personal ideological convictions" (2017, 239), it seems that they have missed something very important about the phenomenon of conscientious objection. The reality is that many if not most cases of conscientious objection are concerned with the goods of medical practice, *not* personal values that are alien to medicine. Claiming that all appeals to conscience are "ideological" is misguided at best and deceptive and tendentious at worst.[10]

With this in mind, we should give physicians latitude to practise in accord with their considered judgements just as we give physicians latitude in clinical practice generally to practise in a manner consistent with their best clinical and moral insights. Conscientious objection – understood as a disagreement about the goods of healthcare – is not concerned with arbitrary likes and dislikes (Schuklenk and Smalling 2017, 238). Rather, it is about a physician's legitimate exercise of the independent moral and technical judgement concerning how best to realise the goods of healthcare. When a junior neonatologist comes to a considered view about the immorality of the withdrawal of treatment from otherwise viable neonates, for example, we should respect that clinician's viewpoint rather than attempting to restrict their right to conscientious objection and forcing them to withdraw treatment from babies when they are directed to do so by a senior clinician. There is nothing manifestly ideological about this kind of dissensus in clinical practice. Indeed, it is congruent with the telos of medicine.

Critics of conscientious objection focus their attack on conscientious objection to socially divisive medical practices such as an abortion, euthanasia and emergency contraception. Yet in many cases the content of physicians' objections to these procedures is no different to objections that one might otherwise describe as purely technical disagreements (for example, disagreements about whether another round of chemotherapy is clinically advisable for a terminally ill patient, or objections to the prescription of a drug treatment like Remdezivir for severe COVID-19 for which there is limited clinical evidence). Doctors' objections to abortion or euthanasia are often based on a conception of what constitutes good medical practice. The claim that conscientious objectors make with respect to abortion or euthanasia is that taking life is not part of good medical practice. It would be a mistake to attempt to categorically distinguish this from other exercises of physician discretion that form part of routine medical practice. While abortion and euthanasia are social divisive practices, this does not mean that the reasons for physicians' objections to these practices are ideological in nature. On the contrary, objecting physicians argue that these practices fall outside of the ambit of good medical practice.

In summary, many if not most instances of conscientious objection in medicine can be characterised as NoMCOs (Kim and Ferguson 2021). That is to say, the physician's conscientious objection is underpinned by a particular conception of what constitutes good medical care. As such, we should not view conscientious objection as involving an imposition of personal values on patients. Rather, we should recognise the integral role that physician discretion plays in the cultivation of virtue and character. There are, of course, limits to what might be considered a reasonable conscientious objection that ought to be accommodated in medicine. It is to this topic that I now turn.

3. Reasonable disagreement about the nature of healthcare

I have argued that we ought to allow doctors to practise in accord with their understanding of what constitutes good medical practice. That is to say, we should permit disagreements among physicians about the nature of medicine and how one ought to go about realising the goals of medicine (Saad 2019; Kim and Ferguson 2021). There are, however, certain limits to what might be considered a reasonable conception of medical practice. First, we should remember that we have ruled out from our study of conscientious objection both a mere dereliction of duty on the part of healthcare practitioners and objections based on social prejudice of one kind or another. We are assuming, then, that we are dealing with physicians who are legitimately trying to get to the truth of what constitutes good medical care. We are not concerned with physicians who are neglecting their duties or who are racist, sexist or otherwise prejudiced in their views of patients. This kind of conduct should not be identified with conscientious objection; rather, physicians who act in this way ought to be sanctioned by the profession. Objections that are clearly based on prejudice have no place in contemporary medical practice and should be disallowed.

But it is also necessary to offer an account of reasonableness and to put forward some criteria for assessing the reasonableness of a conscientious objection. The following two subsections will undertake these tasks.

Reasonableness

Many theorists propose that we employ a standard of reasonableness when assessing the validity of conscientious objections. There is significant disagreement about what a reasonableness test means, but many scholars associate the idea of reasonableness with basic standards of decency and reciprocity in ethics.

Specifically, scholars argue that conscientious objection ought to be permitted provided it does not do harm to others and provided that it is based upon moral reasons that are intelligible to the average person. Wicclair, for example, defends a policy of reasonable accommodation of conscientious objection based on an objection's compatibility with the core values of Western medicine (2019, 561). He also argues that objections cannot be based on invidious discrimination or demonstrably false clinical beliefs (2019, 561).

One common criticism of conscientious objection provisions, however, is that it is impossible to draw a principled distinction between conscientious objections that are permissible and reasonable and conscientious objections that are beyond the pale of reasonableness. Indeed, it could be argued that the concept of *reasonableness* itself is dubious and should not be relied on in the conscientious objection debate. Giubilini and Savulescu (2018), for example, have raised this criticism of conscience protections based on a "reasonableness test":

> [W]hat is "reasonable"? In one broad sense of "reasonable", you can find at least one reasonable person who would object to pretty much any activity that falls within professional standards and expectations. . . . The fact that John Rawls himself was reluctant to provide a definition of "reasonable" and more often relied on what he took to be an intuitive sense of the term is quite telling of how fishy the concept is.

With this in mind, one could argue that we should be deeply suspicious of attempts to rely on a reasonableness test to distinguish legitimate conscientious objections from impermissible objections. A reasonableness test could be seen as a dubious way to avoid addressing an inherent ambiguity in the way we distinguish permissible conscientious objections from impermissible ones (Giubilini 2017).

I am significantly less pessimistic about a reasonableness test and its ability to distinguish permissible from impermissible conscientious objections. Reasonableness is an idea that is deeply embedded in anglophone culture, and common law practitioners have spent centuries defining and refining the criteria on which reasonableness tests are based (Wierzbicka 2006, 104–137). There is a very sophisticated jurisprudence surrounding the definition of reasonableness and how this concept relates to other concepts like rationality, prudential judgement and community standards. It would be misleading to suggest that an appeal to a notion of reasonableness was just a ruse to avoid addressing other difficult questions. This is not to say that there isn't ambiguity surrounding the application of the concept to margin cases; it is true that in at least some legal cases there is robust dispute about whether someone can be deemed to have acted reasonably in a particular situation. Yet the fact that it is difficult to tell where the boundary of reasonableness lies is not to the point: that is true of "grey" as well without there being anything wrong with the concept of grey. The concept of reasonableness is open-textured, but this is not a reason to abandon it.

Some critics, nevertheless, argue that the concept of reasonableness lacks any meaningful content. One plausible criterion for the reasonableness of a conscientious objection, however, would be whether a conscientious objection falls within the bounds of what might be considered a coherent conception of medicine. That is to say, we should consider whether a conscientious objection can plausibly be characterised as a rational concern about how we ought best to realise the goods of medicine in a particular situation. Indeed, it seems that the reasons for allowing at least some scope for conscientious objection are similar to the reasons why we permit professional dissensus in medicine generally (Wilkinson, Truog and Savulescu 2016). Conscientious objection may in fact shed light on the fallibility of an existing professional consensus vis-à-vis the permissibility of morally contentious medical practices. Admittedly, there will always still be some ambiguity surrounding the way in which we distinguish permissible from impermissible conscientious objections. But then again, we should be careful about demanding a kind of certitude that practical ethics as a discipline is unable to yield. As Aristotle (1952) writes in *The Nicomachean Ethics*,

> a well-schooled man is one who searches for that degree of precision in each kind of study which the nature of the subject at hand admits: it is obviously just as foolish to accept arguments of probability from a mathematician as to demand strict demonstrations from an orator.

Some criteria for reasonableness

This subsection will consider a series of criteria according to which a conscientious objection can be considered *reasonable* or *unreasonable*. By *reasonable*, I have in mind whether a conscientious objection is coherent in both its nature and content and when it is weighed against other competing moral considerations that might conflict with permitting conscientious objection. This section will be divided into two subsections – *intrinsic factors* and *extrinsic factors* – that are relevant to assessing the reasonableness of a conscientious objection.

By way of clarification, I am not hereby endorsing some disguised form of conscience tribunal in which objectors must make the case as to whether they fulfil the criteria outlined in this section. Rather, my intention is to outline general characteristics of permissible forms of conscientious objection that can in turn be reflected in whatever administrative mechanisms health authorities choose to adopt for accommodating conscientious objection in the workplace. In the following chapter I will argue against conscience tribunals that place the burden of proof on conscientious objectors. The criteria outlined later, however, might otherwise be reflected in the content of clinical guidelines or relevant legislation governing conscientious objection.

Intrinsic factors

There are several intrinsic factors that we might consider relevant to assessing the reasonableness of a conscientious objection. In this section I will focus on two in particular: the compatibility of an objection with current knowledge in medicine and science and the requirement that an objection be to a procedure and not to a characteristic of patients.

COMPATIBILITY WITH CURRENT KNOWLEDGE IN MEDICINE AND SCIENCE

It is fair to expect that a conscientious objection – insofar as it falls within the category of Nature of Medicine Conscientious Objections (NoMCOs) (Kim and Ferguson 2021) – is based on accurate empirical beliefs about medicine. That is to say, a grounding belief must be consonant with relevant empirical data (and within the bounds of academic interpretation of that data) drawn from basic science and the field of medicine (Card 2014). Suppose, for example, that a physician conscientiously objects to prescribing pain medications since s/he believes that patients do not "really' feel pain. Even though philosophical puzzles persist regarding the existence of pain in others, it is difficult to imagine a provider meeting the burden of proof of reasonability such that she could receive an exemption on the basis of this reason.[11]

Alternatively, we might consider the less-fanciful example of a doctor who declares that they have a conscientious objection to administering vaccines during a pandemic. It may be that the doctor wrongly believes that government-approved vaccines are dangerously unsafe and should not be in general use. If indeed the doctor's beliefs are solely based on conspiracy theories and have no grounding in science, then it is difficult to see why we should permit conscientious objection in this case. Unless a clinician can produce substantial scientific evidence as to the dangers inherent in vaccine use for the general population, then it is difficult to see why we should permit them to opt out of what might otherwise be considered a basic duty for them (particularly when time is of the essence in a pandemic vaccination programme).[12]

OBJECTIONS MUST BE TO PROCEDURES AND NOT TO CLASSES OF A PATIENTS

Of particular importance, a justified conscientious objection must not be concerned with a category of patient but rather must be to a procedure or practice. A clinician should not be afforded the right to conscientiously object to providing medical treatment to particular minorities in society (for example, particular ethnic groups, people of a particular religion, women or members LGBTQI+ community). To invoke a Rawlsian account of reasonableness, medical practitioners ought to be "willing to govern [their] conduct by a principle of equity" (Sibley 1953, 560). If indeed conscientious objectors seek respect for their personal views about the morality of particular procedures, they should not in turn refuse to provide healthcare for particular classes of patients.

Admittedly, this criterion may be more controversial where we are dealing with religious objections. For example, a Muslim medical practitioner might object to conducting intimate physical examinations on patients of the opposite sex (Strickland 2012). But religious objections can and should be subject to the same standards of justification as non-religious objections. In particular, conscientious objectors with a religious objection that discriminates against minority groups in society should not be allowed to opt out of the provision of care for members of the minority groups in question. It is the responsibility of a healthcare professional to provide care for all people in need of it; one cannot discriminate against particular persons (even if discrimination is supposedly sanctioned by one's religion). Furthermore, one cannot object to a procedure based on manifestly inaccurate beliefs about the procedure in question.

Extrinsic factors

It is also apposite here to consider extrinsic factors that might be relevant to the tolerance of conscientious objection. To do this, we should consider what the basic meaning of conscientious objection provisions is intended to be. Conscience provisions are not intended to provide conscientious objectors with a platform for subverting existing laws or disrupting the provision of services that some clinicians might deem to be morally problematic. Conscience protections, rather, are intended to be a way in which we can respect the considered judgements of doctors qua moral agents. In light of this, doctors should not attempt to wield their right to conscientious objection as a means to disrupt medical care or to undermine respect for the rule of law.

One might argue that there are circumstances in which conscientious objection can legitimately be disruptive of the medical system, such as in situations of manifest social injustice (Pruski 2020). I would not dispute the substance of this claim, but I would question the language in which it is couched. I would argue that it may be more fitting to use the label "civil disobedience" to describe this kind of objection. I do not, however, have space here to defend this claim at length. Suffice to say that civil disobedience has an essential orientation towards the disruption of government power or government mandates, whereas conscientious objection is, for our purposes, something more focused on acting in accord with one's own considered moral judgements.

THE WEAPONISATION OF CONSCIENCE

It may be the case that a doctor not only objects to a procedure but acts in a manner that is disruptive to the hospital or medical clinic performing the procedure. It could be that the doctor engages in sabotage to prevent his hospital unit from providing particular services or deliberately sidelines other clinicians who might not share their objection. This behaviour goes beyond one's right to conscientious objection and would not be protected by relevant conscience provisions as envisaged by them.

The case of the Glasgow Midwives discussed in Chapter 1 is interesting to consider in this context. I would argue that the midwives were *not* in fact engaged in act of deliberate sabotage of services even though they did refuse to roster on staff to perform abortions assigned to their hospital unit. The primary intention of the nurses was not to prevent the hospital from providing any abortions. Rather, their concern was to act in accord with their deeply held moral beliefs in situations where they were being asked to do something immoral. If the nurses had engaged in a more far-reaching disruption of services then perhaps one could say they had weaponised the right to conscientious objection. As it stands, however, it seems that the nurses were simply seeking to act in accord with their deeply held beliefs concerning abortion.

Alta Charo (2005) has discussed in particular issues pertaining to clinicians who seek to exercise their right to conscientious objection while holding monopolistic control over a medical resource. If indeed a doctor is seeking to undermine the enactment of the law through deliberately impeding the provision of controversial medical services, then perhaps their right to conscientious objection should be subject to certain restrictions. At the very least, one ought to make known to relevant authorities that one is a conscientious objector and that one cannot provide the service in question, thus allowing the state to seek to make alternative provisions for ensuring that patients can access the service in question. Charo writes:

> Claiming an unfettered right to personal autonomy while holding monopolistic control over a public good constitutes an abuse of the public trust – all the worse if it is not in fact a personal act of conscience but, rather, an attempt at cultural conquest.

> (Charo 2005, 2473)

While I would not go so far as to say that conscientious objection in rural or remote areas – the locations that Charo has in mind – is illicit, I would agree with her that some degree of compromise is required whereby objecting clinicians seek to not impede the provision of the contentious service in question to patients. By the same token, however, the onus should not be on conscientious objectors to make up for the lack of access to morally contentious services like abortion in rural areas. This is ultimately the state's responsibility, as it is the state who is committed to making these services universally available.

SHAMING AND CENSURING PATIENTS

Doctors must also be careful in the way that they make their objections known to patients. Patients should not be made to feel guilty or ashamed for requesting services that are safe and legal. Doctors are more than welcome to explain their reasons as to why they have a moral objection to the procedure in question, yet this right would not go so far as to allow doctors to morally chastise patients. This would be an abuse of the power differential that exists between doctors and patients. It would run afoul of a doctor's fiduciary commitments to patients. Indeed, it would be a sign of vice rather than an exercise of virtue. Rather, doctors should simply make known their objection and release a patient from their care.

There may be cases where patients take subjective offence at the fact that a doctor has a conscientious objection to the procedure that they request. A patient's subjective offence at the actions of the doctor should not be confused with the reality of a doctor's bearing and behaviour. It would only be in cases where a doctor accuses a patient of wrongdoing, moral failing or weakness where we might say that a doctor has veered into the territory of shaming a patient. A looser definition of this criterion could lead to the disallowing of most conscientious objections, as it is not unlikely that a patient will take offence when their treating doctor declares that they have a conscientious objection to a requested service.

Summary

Earlier in this chapter I argued that we ought to permit conscientious objections at least insofar as they are underpinned by disagreements about the nature of medicine. In this section I have outlined a principle of reasonableness that can be used to circumscribe the limits of what we might consider reasonable disagreement about the nature of medicine. I am significantly less pessimistic than other commentators about the ability of a notion of reasonableness to allow us to distinguish between legitimate forms of conscientious objection that ought to be permitted and other forms of objection that ought not to be allowed. The practical criteria I have outlined are some of the more salient criteria that might be employed to determine if an objection ought to be permitted.

Conclusion

In this chapter I have argued in favour of a broad right of conscientious objection for medical professionals. Certain discretionary freedoms are necessary if clinicians are to be able to cultivate the character traits and virtues that we take to be essential for excellence in medical practice. Without the freedom to form one's own view of the nature of good medicine, clinicians will not acquire the character traits that we take to be constitutive of virtue in medical practice. Rather, they will be governed by an ethic of compliance based on external moral norms. This ethic is opposed to an authentic medical professionalism and would be harmful to not only individual practitioners but also the ability of medicine to perform its role in society (Arthur *et al.* 2015). This chapter concluded with a discussion of the conditions under which a conscientious objection can be considered *reasonable*. This chapter has, however, been largely theoretical in character. In the next chapter, we will look more specifically at the laws and professional regulations that govern conscientious objection in medicine. I will consider how conscientious objection should be accommodated in medical practice. I will argue against legal frameworks and healthcare that attempt to stifle the exercise of conscience by placing extensive limits on the grounds deemed to be permissible for conscientious objection. I will also consider how conscientious objectors might be accommodated through registers and doctor-patient matching.

Notes

1 It is worth noting that healthcare professions in countries such as the United Kingdom have training on reflective practice for students and experienced healthcare practitioners. See, for example, General Medical Council. *The Reflective Medical Practitioner: Guidance for Doctors and Medical Students*. London: General Medical Council, 2021; Royal College of Nursing. "Revalidation requirements: Reflection and reflective discussion". London: Royal College of Nursing, 2021. Available from www.rcn.org.uk/professional-development/revalidation/reflection-and-reflective-discussion.

2 Xenomelia, literally meaning "foreign limb", is a neuropsychiatric condition in which nonpsychotic individuals have an intense, persistent belief that one or more of their limbs does not belong to their body; instead they regard it as an alien appendage that should be discarded.

3 Some bioethicists, however, defend the morality of these practices. See, for example, David Oderberg. *Applied Ethics: A Non-Consequentialist Approach*. London: Blackwell, 2004: Ch. 4; Julian Savulescu, Bennett Foddy, John Rogers. "Why we should allow performance enhancing drugs in sport". *British Journal of Sports Medicine* 38 (2004): 666–674.

4 By "the relief of suffering" I have in mind the relief of suffering related to illness and injury. There are some forms of suffering such as loneliness or moral suffering that may fall outside the remit of medicine.

5 There are some scholars who offer a much richer, theological conception of the nature of medical practice and conceive of medicine as existing in fruitful partnership with the great spiritual traditions of the world. For more on this view of medicine, see Michael and Tracey Balboni. *Hostility to Hospitality: Spirituality and Professional Socialisation in Medicine*. New York: Oxford University Press, 2018. I do not mean to foreclose the possibility that medicine can exist in a fruitful, symbiotic relationship with religious and spiritual traditions. To discuss this possibility in depth, however, would be beyond the scope of this book.

6 Note that in many legal jurisdictions malpractice is judged in part by the opinions of expert witnesses who are ultimately one's professional peers. That is to say, "the specific duty owed by the physician to the patient is defined by the profession itself" (Bal 2009, 383).

7 The Tuskegee Study of Untreated Syphilis in the Negro Male was an ethically abusive study conducted between 1932 and 1972 by the United States Public Health Service and the Centers for Disease Control and Prevention on a group of nearly 400 African Americans with syphilis. The purpose of the study was to observe the effects of the disease when untreated, though by the end of the study it was entirely treatable. The men were not informed of the nature of the experiment, and more than 100 died as a result.

8 In a survey of 549 doctors and medical students, Arthur *et al.* (2015, 31) found that "in explaining their thinking about ethical medical practice, experienced doctors were more likely to rely on their judgement, while those at earlier career stages were more likely to rely on rules". This finding echoes my contention that virtuous medical practitioners are those who possess a refined capacity for clinical judgement, as opposed to a rigid, rule-bookish approach to medical decision-making.

9 For an account of what distinguishes a profession from other forms of work, see Sulmasy (2017).

10 Note that most scholars agree that conscientious objection ought to be permitted in circumstances where it is necessary to fight systemic injustice. See Michal Pruski. "Conscientious objection and systemic injustice". *Clinical Ethics* 15:3 (2020): 120–125. There seems to be inconsistency, then, in the criticisms that scholars like Schuklenk and Smalling make about conscientious objection to abortion, euthanasia and other socially contentious medical practices.

11 This example is found in Card (2014, 323).
12 This is not to say that there are no circumstances in which conscientious objection to administering or receiving the COVID-19 vaccine would be legitimate. See Michal Pruski. "Conscience and vaccines: lessons from Babylon-5 and COVID-19". *The New Bioethics* published online 6th August 2021. DOI: doi.org/10.1080/20502877.2021.19 59789.

References

Allen, H. Christine, Garbe, M. Connor, Lees, Julian *et al.* "Off-label medication use in children, more common than we think: A systematic review of the literature". *Journal of the Oklahoma State Medical Association* 111 (2018): 776–783.

Aristotle. *The Works of Aristotle.* W.D. Ross (trans.). Oxford: Clarendon, 1952.

Arthur, James, Kristjansson, Kristjan, Thomas, Hywel *et al. Virtuous Medical Practice.* Birmingham: Jubilee Centre for Character and Virtues, 2015.

Australian Medical Association. *AMA Position Statement on Medical Professionalism.* Sydney: Australian Medical Association, 2010.

Baker, Robert. "The American Medical Association and race". *American Medical Association Journal of Ethics* 14;6 (2014): 479–488.

Bal, Sonny. "The expert witness in medical malpractice litigation". *Clinical Orthopaedics and Related Research* 467 (2009): 383–391.

Balboni, Michael, and Balboni, Tracey. *Hostility to Hospitality: Spirituality and Professional Socialisation in Medicine.* New York: Oxford University Press, 2018.

Biggar, Nigel. "Why religion deserves a place in secular medicine". *Journal of Medical Ethics* 41 (2015): 229–233.

Bott, Elizabeth, Duffy, Ryan, Borges, Nicholas *et al.* "Called to medicine: Physicians experiences of career calling". *The Career Development Quarterly* 65 (2017): 113–130.

Card, Robert. "Reasonability and conscientious objection in medicine: A reply to Marsh and an elaboration of the reason-giving requirement". *Bioethics* 26;6 (2014): 320–326.

Catholic Church. *Catechism of the Catholic Church.* Vatican City: Liberia Editrice Vaticana, 1992.

Cavanaugh, Thomas. *Hippocrates' Oath and Asclepius' Snake.* New York: Oxford University Press, 2018.

Charo, Alta. "The celestial fire of conscience: Refusing to deliver medical care". *New England Journal of Medicine* 352 (2005): 2471–2473.

Cruess, Richard, Cruess, Sylvia, and Steinert, Yvonne. "Medicine as a community of practice: Implications for medical education". *Academic Medicine* 93;2 (2018): 185–191.

Curlin, Farr, and Tollefsen, Christopher. *The Way of Medicine: Ethics and the Healing Professions.* South Bend: University of Notre Dame Press, 2021.Earp, Brian. "Does religion deserve a place in secular medicine?". *Journal of Medical Ethics* 41 (2015): 865–866.

Curlin, Farr, and Tollefsen, Christopher. "Conscience and the way of medicine". *Perspectives in Biology and Medicine* 62;3 (2019): 560–575.

Gamble, Nathan, and Pruski, Michal. "Medical acts and conscientious objection: What can a physician be compelled to do?". *The New Bioethics* 25 (2019): 262–282.

Garcia, Jorge L.A. "Virtues and principles in biomedical ethics". *Journal of Medicine and Philosophy* 29 (2020): 471–503.

General Medical Council. *The Reflective Medical Practitioner: Guidance for Doctors and Medical Students.* London: General Medical Council, 2021.

Giubilini, Alberto. "Objection to conscience: An argument against conscience exemptions in healthcare". *Bioethics* 31;5 (2017): 400–408.

Giubilini, Alberto, and Savulescu, Julian. "Against conscientious objection: A counter-declaration and reply to Oderberg". *Practical Ethics Blog* 11th October 2018.

Hawking, Michael, Curlin, Farr, and Yoon, John. "Courage and compassion: Virtues in caring for so-called difficult patients". *AMA Journal of Ethics* 19;4 (2017): 357–363.

Hong, Angela, Fogarty, Gerald, Dolven-Jacobsen, Kari *et al.* "Adjuvant whole-brain radiation therapy compared with observation after local treatment of melanoma brain metastases: A multicenter, randomized phase III trial". *Journal of Clinical Oncology* 37;33 (2019): 3132–3141.

Keogh, Louise, Gillam, Lynn, Bismark, Marie, *et al.* "Conscientious objection to abortion, the law and its implementation in Victoria, Australia: Perspectives of abortion service providers". *BMC Medical Ethics* 20;11 (2019): 1–10.

Kim, Eric, and Ferguson, Kyle. "Conscientious objection, the nature of medicine, and the need for reformability". *Bioethics* first published 31st August 2021. doi: 10.1111/bioe.12943.

Kyle, Robert, Steensma, David, Shampo, Marc *et al.* "Barry James Marshall – discovery of helicobacter pylori as a cause of peptic ulcer". *Mayo Clinic Proceedings* 91 (2016): 67–68.

LaFollette, Eva, and LaFollette, Hugh. "Private conscience, public acts". *Journal of Medical Ethics* 33;5 (2007): 249–254.

MacIntyre, Alasdair. *After Virtue* (2nd ed.). Notre Dame University Press, 1997.

Makary, Marty. "Surgeon: What they don't teach you in med school". *Time Magazine* 10th January 2014. Available from https://time.com/3268/surgeon-what-they-dont-teach-in-med-school/.

Mill, John Stuart. *On Liberty*. Harlow: Pearson Longman, 2007.

Miller, Frank, Brody, Howard, and Cheng, Kevin. "Cosmetic surgery and the internal morality of medicine". *Cambridge Quarterly of Healthcare Ethics* 9 (2000): 353–364.

Miller, Franklin G., and Brody, Howard. "The internal morality of medicine: An evolutionary perspective". *Journal of Medicine and Philosophy* 26 (2001): 581–599.

Minerva, Francesca. "Conscientious objection in Italy". *Journal of Medical Ethics* 41 (2015): 170–173.

Oderberg, David. "The conscientious objection (medical activities) bill: Some objections rebutted". *Journal of Medical Ethics Blog* 16th March 2018.

Pellegrino, Edmund, and Thomasma, David. *The Virtues in Medical Practice*. New York: Oxford University Press, 1993.

Pellegrino, Edmund, and Thomasma, David. *The Christian Virtues in Medical Practice*. Washington, DC: Georgetown University Press, 1996.

Pruski, Michal. "Conscientious objection and systemic injustice". *Clinical Ethics* 15;3 (2020): 120–125.

Pruski, Michal. "Conscience and vaccines: Lessons from Babylon-5 and COVID-19". *The New Bioethics*. Published online 6th August 2021. doi: 10.1080/20502877.2021.1959789.

Royal College of Nursing. "Revalidation requirements: Reflection and reflective discussion". London: Royal College of Nursing, 2021. Available from www.rcn.org.uk/professional-development/revalidation/reflection-and-reflective-discussion.

Saad, Toni. "Conscientious objection and clinical judgement: The right to refuse harm". *The New Bioethics* 25 (2019): 248–261.

Savulescu, Julian. "Conscientious objection in medicine". *British Medical Journal* 332 (2006): 294.

Savulescu, Julian. "Should doctors feel able to practice according to their personal values and beliefs". *Medical Journal of Australia* 195 (2011). doi: 10.5694/mja11.11249.

Savulescu, Julian, and Schuklenk, Udo. "Doctors have no right to refuse medical assistance in dying, abortion or contraception". *Bioethics* 31;3 (2017): 162–170.

Schuklenk, Udo and Smalling, Ricardo. "Why medical professionals have no moral claim to conscientious objection accommodation in liberal democracies". *Journal of Medical Ethics* 43 (2017): 234–240.

Sibley, W.M. "The rational vs. the reasonable". *Philosophical Review* 62 (1953): 554–560.

Stahl, Ronit, and Emanuel, Ezekiel. "Physicians not conscripts: Conscientious objection in healthcare". *New England Journal of Medicine* 376;14 (2017): 1380–1385; 1382.

Strickland, Sophie. "Conscientious objection in medical students: A questionnaire survey". *Journal of Medical Ethics* 38 (2012): 22–25.

Sulmasy, Daniel. "Informed consent without autonomy". *Fordham Urban Law Journal* 30;1 (2002): 207–220.

Sulmasy, Daniel. "'Advance directives' as an extension of the tradition of foregoing extraordinary means of care". *Bioethics Outlook* 19;2 (2008): 1–12.

Sulmasy, Daniel. "Tolerance, professional judgement, and the discretionary space of the physician". *Cambridge Quarterly of Healthcare Ethics* 21;6 (2017): 18–31.

Symons, Xavier. "Pellegrino, MacIntyre, and the internal morality of clinical medicine". *Theoretical Medicine and Bioethics* 40;3 (2019): 243–251.

Veatch, Robert. "The impossibility of a morality internal to Medicine". *Journal of Medicine and Philosophy* 26 (2001): 621–642.

Weinstock, Daniel. "Conscientious refusal and health professionals: Does religion make a difference". *Bioethics* 28;1 (2014): 8–15.

Wicclair, Mark. "Preventing conscientious objection in medicine from running amok: A defense of reasonable accommodation". 40;6 (2019): 539–564.

Wierzbicka, Anna. *English: Meaning and Culture*. London: Oxford University Press, 2006.

Wilkinson, Dominic. "Conscientious non-objection in intensive care". *Cambridge Quarterly of Healthcare Ethics* 26;1 (2017): 132–142.

Wilkinson, Dominic, Truog, Robert, and Savulescu, Julian. "In favour of medical dissensus: Why we should agree to disagree about end-of-life decisions". *Bioethics* 30;2 (2016): 109–118.

World Health Organisation. *Basic Documents* (49th ed.). Geneva: World Health Organisation, 2020.

5   Making space for the exercise of conscience in medicine

Introduction

This book has provided a robust moral psychological account of conscience and has argued for the centrality of conscience in medical practice. I do not wish to focus extensively on the practicality of accommodating conscience and conscientious objection in healthcare, if only because this would take us beyond the primary aims of the book. The accommodation of conscientious objection, furthermore, is to some extent contingent on the specific features of different healthcare settings, such as the nature of a healthcare system, the nature of the legal and regulatory frameworks by which it is governed, and the availability of alternative service options for patients. For this reason, I will not provide a detailed, practical model of how we ought to accommodate conscientious objection. I will, nevertheless, engage with recent proposals in the literature on conscientious objection and will consider the extent to which healthcare regulators might address some of the key issues of conflict that potentially arise with conscientious objection.

Section 1 offers a critical evaluation of recent proposals for the regulation of conscientious objection in healthcare, including the idea of a blanket ban, conscience tribunals and referral requirements. Section 2 of this chapter provides some general suggestions for how we might accommodate conscientious objectors in healthcare. I focus in particular on a public register for conscientious objectors, conscientious objection quotas and a system of doctor-patient matching.

1. A critical evaluation of recent proposals for the regulation of conscientious objection

Several proposals for regulating conscientious objection have featured in recent bioethics literature. In this section, I will discuss three of the most prominent proposals. The first of these is that we should introduce a blanket ban on conscientious objection in healthcare practice. Stahl and Emanuel and Savulescu and Schuklenk suggest that conscientious objectors ought to comply with existing professional standards, or, alternatively, they should leave the medical profession (Stahl and Emanuel 2017; Savulescu and Schuklenk 2017). The second proposal is that we should introduce conscience tribunals, whereby healthcare professionals

DOI: 10.4324/9781003247623-5

are required to justify, to the satisfaction of a board of arbitration, that they should be afforded the right to conscientious objection (Card 2017; Clarke 2017a). The third proposal concerns referral requirements for healthcare professionals. Specifically, some scholars argue that healthcare professionals with a conscientious objection should be required to refer their patients to a practitioner who, to the best of their knowledge, will be willing to perform the procedure (Cowley 2017; McLeod 2020).

A total ban

Some scholars argue that conscientious objection should not be permitted in healthcare practice. That is to say, healthcare professionals should be prohibited from objecting to participation in healthcare procedures to which they have a moral objection. They should, rather, set their own personal convictions aside and seek to abide by the requirements of their professional role. Proponents of a ban on conscientious objection argue that the primary duty of healthcare professionals is to promote patient welfare (Savulescu 2006; Savulescu and Schuklenk 2017; Stahl and Emanuel 2017). Doctors are not in medicine to promote their own vision of the good or to practise in accord with their own idiosyncratic understanding of what constitutes good medical care. Rather, doctors are in medicine to act in a manner consonant with existing professional standards and practice guidelines. Doctors, furthermore, should seek to fulfil patient preferences by delivering medical care in a timely manner. In light of these considerations, a widely held view has emerged that conscientious objection should be heavily restricted if allowed at all.

Savulescu and Schuklenk argue that conscientious objection should be effectively outlawed, save for very exceptional circumstances (such as if a nurse were directed to force-feed a prisoner on hunger strike) (2017, 167–168). According to the authors, "patient access to care" should be prioritised over the protection of "doctors' idiosyncratic moral convictions with regard to [medical] services" (2017, 163). What matters most is that legal, beneficial, desired services are provided to patients. Medical professionalism is about putting patient preferences ahead of one's own personal and subjective values.

This has very practical implications for the way in which we regulate conscientious objection in medical practice. Savulescu and Schuklenk suggest that we should select students for medical training who are ready and willing to perform the full suite of practices that form part of modern medicine. They write of the need to select candidates for medical schools "who are tolerant, have epistemic responsibility and humility and are willing to accommodate patient values" (2017, 164). Fully qualified medical practitioners, for their part, should comply with the existing medical consensus on what is considered clinically indicated treatment, and this includes the provision of reproductive healthcare and end-of-life care. If indeed a doctor has a conscientious objection, at the very least he must ensure that care of the patient is passed on to a doctor who will be able to provide timely and effective medical care for that individual (a topic to which we will return shortly). Conscientious objectors who compromise the care of their patients must be disciplined. As Savulescu writes, we risk opening up a Pandora's box of "idiosyncratic, bigoted, discriminatory medicine" if we fail to discipline practitioners who disrupt a patient's access to healthcare (2006, 297).

Stahl and Emanuel offer a similar argument to Savulescu about the practice of conscientious objection. They argue that professional associations should in most cases "resist sanctioning conscientious objection as an acceptable practice" (Stahl and Emanuel 2017, 1380). Professional associations must be given the jurisdiction to determine what is acceptable medical care, and individual practitioners should abide by this. The authors argue that professional associations are in the best epistemic position to identify what contributes to patient well-being and rights. These associations engage in a process of "reflective equilibrium" – a kind of collective dialectic in which persons seek equilibrium between their basic ethical principles and their intuitions about particular cases (Stahl and Emanuel 2017, 1382). This process leads to "consensus but not necessarily unanimity"; yet consensus is sufficient, in the view of these authors, to mandate that all members of the profession abide by the professional principles identified.

Individual practitioners, in contrast, are not well placed to determine what practices are conducive to patient well-being. Individual practitioners are often motivated by religious sentiment when objecting to the provision of a particular procedure, and this is a poor guide for elucidating the limits of "the primary interest" (Stahl and Emanuel 2017, 1382). In any case, an individual practitioner's personal views are subject to much less scrutiny than a professional code of conduct. The latter would be discussed extensively by many healthcare professionals and only implemented following a period of extensive consultation. The former is just a person's own moral view about a particular issue. According to Savulescu and Schuklenk, personal moral views are "by necessity partially arbitrary" (2017, 167) and should not be allowed to function as a guide for medical practice.

Both Savulescu and Schuklenk and Stahl and Emanuel emphasise that doctors are not conscripts and that we should not see restrictions on conscientious objection as being the equivalent of conscripting soldiers into a traumatic war. Doctors are free to join (and also free to leave) the medical profession. Unlike soldiers, their professional vocation is in their own hands. And if they are not ready to perform procedures that are standard practice in medicine, then it makes sense that they consider finding another profession or a role in medicine that does not conflict with their own conscientious beliefs. This is sometimes known as the *get another job* argument (Sulmasy 2017, 22).

In sum, critics argue that doctors have no *right* to be doctors but rather have been given the *privilege* of being doctors. People entering and practising medicine need to be prepared to put their obligations of service before their own personal interests (Savulescu and Schuklenk 2017, 164; Stahl and Emanuel 2017, 1382). Indeed, medicine would be better if it did not have members with idiosyncratic ideas about the universe and who sought to enforce their own moral views on patients (Savulescu and Schuklenk 2017, 168–169).

The total ban view, however, fails to take into account the fact that medicine itself involves a journey of conscience, whereby practitioners must determine what in their considered view constitutes acceptable and ethical medical practice (Curlin and Tollefsen 2021). Doctors must constitute their moral and technical rationality through a process of formation, which will involve listening to their peers and informing oneself of relevant professional guidelines, but that also involves personal discernment and discretion vis-à-vis the practice of medicine. We cannot get rid of conscience from medicine, whether we like it or not. Conscience plays an integral part in the professional formation of doctors. A ban on the exercise of conscience would deny this basic truth of medicine and would potentially impair the moral development of clinicians. We need discerning physicians, not automatons, in our medical clinics and operating theatres.

It also seems misleading to contrast the well-reasoned deliberative democratic processes of professional associations with the fundamentally arbitrary, unreasonable and idiosyncratic personal views of medical practitioners. It is my claim that a reasonable moral agent's convictions of conscience have in fact been sifted through a rigorous critical filter, namely the critical filter of one's professional experiences and one's acquired professional wisdom. To ask someone to renounce a moral truth that they have acquired through their professional experience and sifted through their own capacity for moral reflection is akin to asking someone to say that $2+2$ equals 5. A judgement of conscience is more than just a judgement about personal belief; it's a judgement about how one understands the moral structure of reality. We would then be asking people not only to deny a particular belief but also to deny what, in the last analysis, is the result of their own sincere and intellectually virtuous efforts to know reality. With this in mind, judgements of a considered conscience that meet basic standards of reasonableness ought to be afforded respect even where they come into conflict with professional guidelines.

Why not compromise, however?[1] Critics don't provide a good reason as to why authorities ought not to seek a compromise that respects conscience rights while meeting patient needs. Critics argue that doctors have no right to conscientious objection, but the principle basis for this claim is a contentious account of the nature of medicine and the duties of medical practitioners (and, ultimately, a contested anthropology).[2] We should remember that critics are claiming that conscience rights do not matter at all, not that they matter *less*. Critics of conscientious objection thus set a very high bar and fall well short of refuting the case for conscience rights.

Proponents of a ban on conscientious objection might argue that compromises will not work and that we need a ban to ensure that patients actually get access to the services they need and want. But once again, critics do not do enough to demonstrate that compromises are impracticable. Often their criticism relies on a caricature of conscientious objectors as intransigent ideologues who will stop at nothing short of morally chastising patients for seeking to solicit immoral services. The reality – as I have argued in the previous chapters – is far from this. Rather, conscientious objection in its archetypal form is concerned with a dispute about the proper goals of medicine, the nature of therapy and the moral appropriateness of treatment in a particular situation. It's not an issue of physicians imposing their views on patients; it's about physicians acting in accord with their considering understanding of good medical practice. It would be unfair to characterise this kind of situation as an instance of bigotry.

Critics of conscientious objection are also concerned about the risk that conscience provisions could sanction idiosyncratic medical practice. Yet they do not do enough to demonstrate the seriousness of this risk, either. Savulescu makes a cautionary comment about the risk of "opening a pandora's box of idiosyncratic medicine", but we do not know if this is borne out by reality. The fact that the literature on conscientious objection and disruption of service is largely anecdotal would seem to give us some reason to suspect that the concerns raised by conscientious objectors are inadequately substantiated. A widely cited study by Keogh *et al.* (2019) on the impact of conscientious objection to abortion, for example, relies on interviews with abortion providers rather than conscientious objectors themselves. The authors also note that their study "[does] not give any indication as to the size of the problem" (2019, 8).

Conscience tribunals

Other scholars have argued that we should introduce conscience tribunals for healthcare professionals, whereby healthcare providers and healthcare authorities are authorised to take disciplinary action against doctors who disrupt the provision of care through their conscientious non-participation (Clarke 2017a, 2017b; Hughes 2017). The basic proposal is that a tribunal be established for the purposes of determining whether conscientious objectors should be allowed to opt out of participation in certain medical procedures. The tribunal would be constituted of a mix of healthcare professionals and state representatives who could together assess the validity of individual conscience claims. Objecting healthcare professionals would be required to demonstrate, to the satisfaction of the panel, that their conscientious objection is sincere, rational and not unduly obstructive of efficient and timely medical care for patients.

One insight motivating this proposal is the notion that conscientious objectors should have reasonable grounds for opting out of what would otherwise be considered to be a routine part of their own professional duties. Doctors should not be able to opt out of their professional work just because they find it unappealing or unpalatable or problematic for some other non-serious reason. Rather, they should provide an argument as to why the practice in question conflicts with their long-standing and deeply held personal beliefs and why these beliefs are deserving of respect. They should also have to demonstrate that their refusal of care "is compatible with unimpeded access to [medical] services by patients" (Hughes 2017, 217). A panel of clinicians and public servants are in a good position to assess whether these criteria have been met.

Proponents of tribunals also rely heavily on the use of a military analogy for conscientious objection in medicine (Clarke 2017a, 2017b). It is true that doctors are not like conscripted soldiers. They have not been co-opted to fight in battle. Yet precisely for this reason they should have to justify why their own non-participation in routine medical procedures ought to be tolerated in the medical system. Currently, medical practitioners in many jurisdictions are given broad scope to practise in accord with their deeply held beliefs, and they are not required to justify their practices in any way. A tribunal would be a reasoned compromise between allowing an unfettered right to conscientious objection and banning the practice all together.

The burden of proof in the proposed tribunals lies with conscientious objectors. Conscientious objectors would need to justify why they should be allowed to opt out of participation in the problematic procedures in question. Doctors are ordinarily expected to comply with their professional duties, and so conscientious objection should be "an exception rather than routine practice" (Hughes 2017, 216). Conscientious objectors ought to explain why they should be granted an exemption from their ordinary professional responsibilities.

One function of conscience tribunals, according to Steve Clarke, is to determine what alternative medical service objecting practitioners ought to be expected to provide (or – if their justification for their conscientious objection is bad – whether they should be directed to seek employment elsewhere) (2017a, 219–220). Clarke suggests that doctors who object to abortion but do not object to working for an organisation that provides abortion are rationally inconsistent. They should be encouraged to find work in an organisation that is less at odds with their own personal values. Part of the role of the tribunal is to help them to see why they are misguided in their manner of rationalising their actions (2017a, 219).

The idea of conscience tribunals may strike many as a means of compromising on the contentious question of how to regulate conscientious objection. It could be argued that we should allow some forms of conscientious objection, but – as we stated earlier – objecting physicians ought to be prepared to justify themselves to their peers and relevant authorities and to explain why they ought to be given the right to conscientious objection. This could be seen as getting the balance right between tolerating conscientious objection on the one hand and ensuring patients get access to medical services in a timely fashion on the other.

Conscientious objectors should not, however, have to justify their actions to a tribunal as if they were suspected of committing a crime. To act in accord with one's conscience is a moral virtue rather than a sign of a warped moral psychology. Conscience, furthermore, is integral to medical practice, and respect for conscience is a fundamental principle of medicine. Allowing physicians to act in accord with their own reasonable conception of good medical practice is an essential part of the cultivation of virtue and character in medicine. With this in mind, we should not put the burden of proof on conscientiously objecting doctors to justify to a tribunal why they should have their beliefs respected. Deference to authority and rule-following is, in some cases, of the utmost importance in medicine. Yet this does not give health authorities license to treat conscientious objectors as rule-breakers.

We should bear in mind the symbolic meaning that conscience tribunals carry, particularly in light of the historical use of conscientious objection tribunals in the military. As Kessler (2015, 454) observes, even the more accommodating conscientious objection tribunals in World War I were characterised as "tyrannical" (see also McDermott 2011, 36–58). There was a view among administrators that conscientious objectors were often if not mostly inauthentic and were instead using conscientious objection as an excuse for one to shirk one's patriotic responsibilities. Conscience tribunals, then, bear the subtext that one may be failing to live up to one's professional responsibilities. Conscience tribunals, in other words, are not politically neutral instruments that ensure justice and right conduct. Rather, they have at their core a suspicion of the exercise of conscience and the potentially harmful effects that conscience may have on conduct in the professions.

Consider, furthermore, how members of the public would react if conscience tribunals were set up for the exercise of other fundamental freedoms such as a freedom of expression, freedom of assembly, freedom of association and so forth. The public would be repulsed at the thought of citizens having to justify the exercise of their fundamental rights to a civil tribunal. Why ought the situation to be different for medical doctors? Does membership of the medical profession really imply a suspension of fundamental civil rights?

Granted, it may make sense to provide an avenue of redress in the healthcare system for patients and healthcare providers who claim to have been adversely affected by conscientious objection. A tribunal could be established for these purposes and could review the evidence to determine if indeed it supports restricting a particular clinician's right to conscientious objection. But the emphasis is different in this case, and rightly so. We are not placing the burden of proof on clinicians to show why their conscience-based objection ought to be respected. Rather, we are providing a means by which to address the supposedly deleterious implications that conscientious objection might have for the provision of care. This system does not run afoul of the basic presumption in favour of permitting conscientious objection.

It is appropriate to distinguish my view from the view advanced by Robert Card (2016). Card argues that we should assess a provider's reasons for his or her objection before granting a conscientious exemption. He advocates something akin to a conscience tribunal for resolving these disputes. If the medical professional's reasoned basis involves an empirical mistake, for example, an accommodation is not warranted. A conscientious objection tribunal could ensure that conscientious objectors are not basing their decisions on these sorts of errors. Card also argues for a reasonability standard to be used to assess the validity of a stated justification for conscientious objection. He is supportive of a policy establishing conscientious objector status in medicine.

The difference between Robert Card's thesis and my basic argument, however, is that Card argues that "a conscientious refusal requires a greater burden of proof, all things being equal, as compared to a conscientious provision of care" (Card 2011). That is, Card argues that the burden of proof is on the conscientious objector to justify their objection to the satisfaction of their peers, rather than there being a presumption in favour of the right to conscientious objection. My position, in contrast, is one that avowedly defends the practice of conscientious objection. Unlike Card, I argue that there are a plurality of views on what constitutes good medical practice and that there should be a presumption in favour of the right to conscientiously object (Symons 2019). The onus would be on patients or healthcare providers to demonstrate that conscientious objectors were sufficiently disruptive of services to warrant censure or restrictions. Conscience is integral to medical practice, and there should be a presumption in favour of permitting its exercise.

We also ought not to overlook the pitfalls of determining whether a particular physician has made an empirical mistake in his or her stated justification for a conscience-based exemption. Granted, it may be easy to determine if a physician's beliefs are based on conspiracy theories (such as conspiracies about COVID-19 vaccines). It may be more difficult, however, to assess a claim such as a claim about the psychological impact of abortion on women. One could easily see a process of arbitration becoming politicised where it concerned matters such as "contraindications" for abortion or similarly contentious procedures. If a tribunal of the kind described in the previous paragraph were ever established, there would need to be strong safeguards in place to ensure that it did not turn into a surreptitious means to suppress conscientious objection altogether.

Referral requirements

Another function of conscience tribunals, according to Clarke, is to determine whether a conscientiously objecting doctor should be obliged to refer their patients to practitioners who can provide the service that they are not prepared to provide (2017a, 220). It is to the topic of medical referral that we now turn.

One very common proposal in literature – and, indeed, a common feature of law and policy dealing with conscientious objection – is the requirement that objecting clinicians refer patients to other clinicians who are willing to provide the service in question. If doctors aren't willing to provide a service themselves, they ought to ensure the patient can connect with someone who can. The most common argument in favour of this proposal is that doctors should be willing to compromise when they have a conscientious objection; providing a referral limits the inconvenience and harm caused by a doctor's conscientious objection. In this brief section, I will provide an account of referral requirements and how these referral requirements are philosophically defended.

In medicine, a referral is generally understood as an act whereby a doctor requests that a patient be taken into the care of another physician who can provide them with a service that they require. Referrals are a routine part of medical care that occur once a primary physician (or general practitioner) has seen a patient and determines that they are in need of specialist medical care. We can distinguish what some people called *direct referrals* from a more general provision of information. A direct referral is an act whereby a medical doctor directly requests that another practitioner provide a particular service or set of tests to a patient who is currently in their care. Direct referrals typically take the form of a letter written by the primary physician (or general practitioner) requesting that another physician take the patient into his or her care. The provision of information to a patient, by contrast, might simply involve general information about where medical services might be obtained. Examples of this include the provision of generic fliers or web information about how a patient might access a suite of services relevant to their current situation or perhaps a verbal representation from a doctor about where a patient might be able to access a service. Some theorists such as Clarke (2017a) argue that there are morally relevant differences between direct referrals and the mere provision of information. One might be viewed as direct and formal cooperation in wrongdoing, whereas the other might be viewed as indirect and non-causal cooperation.

A range of philosophical arguments have been marshalled in favour of referral requirements in medicine. McLeod, for example, argues that it is part of an objecting doctor's fiduciary duties that they refer patients to other physicians who can provide the services that they are seeking (McLeod 2020). A doctor who fails to provide a referral for an abortion, for example, would be abandoning their patient (and this would be particularly problematic where the patient does not know how to navigate the healthcare system). Certainly, there are many theorists who construe this as a gross dereliction of professional duty. In some cases, patients cannot access treatment without a referral, and so the doctor becomes an indispensable part of ensuring that the patient is able to access the kind of medical treatment that they want.

Theorists generally contend that it is more important to give patients access to safe, legal and effective healthcare than allowing a conscientious objector to avoid practices that are inconsistent with the demands of his or her conscience. Certainly, respect for conscience should be given some weight, yet the duty to meet patient needs is paramount. Referral requirements ensure that patients can access the services that they desire.

Many commentators see referral requirements as an important part of flexibility in medicine and a check on what we might call *conscience absolutism*. Wicclair argues that conscience should not be given so much weight that it actually interferes with the provision of care for a patient (Wicclair 2014). Referrals are also a way of putting in check the power of doctors to enforce their particular moral views on patients. Alta Charo (2005, 273) warns of the danger of conscientious objection being weaponised for the purposes of "cultural conquest". Doctors should not be allowed to use conscientious objection to impose a particular vision of morality on their patients.

It could be argued that referrals are just a matter of transferring a patient out of one's care (such as when a doctor in a Catholic nursing home authorises an aged care resident to travel to another aged care home so that they may receive MAiD). Even direct referrals need not necessarily be conceived of as formal cooperation in wrongdoing. Indeed, Cowley argues that "proximity is hard to measure, morally" and that even after a referral has been issued, "there are several steps that remain for the patient and other healthcare professionals to take before the principal act is carried" (2017, 209). According to Cowley, the fact that a patient can choose not to act on the information "breaks the chain of cooperation, collapses the putative necessity of the [doctor's] contribution and means that the [doctor's] objection is not morally undermined by her providing the information" (2017, 210). The referring doctor is not causally responsible, in other words, for the patient's choice to procure an abortion.

Doctors who have a conscientious objection, however, should not be required to refer patients for treatment as a direct referral constitutes direct cooperation in wrongdoing. The supposed compromise that referrals involve is not really a compromise at all. A referring doctor is complicit in the act of providing a service to which they have a moral objection. They may not have to perform an immoral act, but they still remain facilitators of the immoral act.

Indeed, both critics and proponents of conscience rights recognise that referral requirements involve a problematic form of complicity in the very act to which a doctor has an objection (Trigg 2017; Clarke 2017a; Savulescu and Schuklenk, 2017). As Steve Clarke (2017a, 220) writes:

> The [referral] expectation is controversial because it causally implicates conscientious objectors with the very act that they conscientiously refuse to provide. If I am convinced that abortion is morally wrong, then by referring a patient to a willing abortion provider I knowingly enable an act to occur that I consider wrong. Surely I bear some causal responsibility for its occurrence.

It is not just casual responsibility, for that matter. Arguably, the doctor has *moral* responsibility for assisting the patient in accessing the service deemed to be objectionable. This would explain why many doctors are loath to accept the supposed compromise. Thus, Savulescu and Schuklenk (2017, 168) write:

> If authorizing an abortion (for example) were really in itself evil (both objectively and significantly immoral), it is hard to see how proposed referral policies could be tenable. If the practice is evil, the individual should not be any part of it, even by being a member of that speciality or profession.

It does not make sense, then, to see referral requirements as a compromise. There may perhaps be some situations where doctors, based on their own moral beliefs, do not see a problem with referring for abortions and only have an objection to performing them. Yet as Savulescu and Schuklenk suggest, if one really thought that abortion was seriously immoral one would want nothing to do with it.

There may be some circumstances in which the provision of generic information about a patient's medical options is permissible. An example might be a doctor who has an objection to euthanasia but who directs a patient seeking access to euthanasia to a government website with information on all end-of-life options. Referring a patient to generic government information does not imply an intention that the patient actually accesses the service in question. As Eberl (2019) suggests, it is "material cooperation" that can be justified given "a proportionately serious reason" (576).

We ought not to conflate the provision of generic information, however, with the supply of specific information about practitioners who will provide the service in question. Cowley (2017) uses the example of a GP in the NHS who is a conscientious objector and who has a patient who is seeking an abortion. The GP in Cowley's example tells the patient to go and visit their colleague down the hall who will "give her what she wants" (210). Cowley claims that the GP in this case "is not morally undermined by providing [the patient with] information" (210). Yet I would contend that the GP's actions in this case may in fact amount to complicity, as the GP is providing the patient with clear and specific information about who will provide them with timely access to an abortion. The GP becomes part of the causal chain leading to an abortion (presuming that the woman chooses to go through with the procedure). The fact that the woman is free to act or refrain from acting on the referral is, in my view, beside the point. The doctor is causally implicated in the procurement of an abortion irrespective of these counterfactual considerations.

To be clear, complicity is diminished by the *kind of assistance* that one provides to a patient in accessing a service to which one has an objection. An *effective referral* is "a referral made in good faith" to a non-objecting, available and accessible alternative healthcare provider (College of Physicians and Surgeons of Ontario 2015). Typically, though not always, this will take the form of a written referral. The key feature of an effective referral is that one practitioner directs a patient to another practitioner who they know will provide the service. The referral is made "with a view to supporting . . . access to care". The provision of an effective referral amounts to morally problematic complicity. The provision of generic information, in contrast, may not amount to formal cooperation (depending on the circumstances). In this case, a doctor has simply provided publicly accessible information about the full suite of medical services that are legally available to a patient. Indeed, it is likely that the patient would have found this information anyway even if the doctor did not provide it. The doctor is not an indispensable link in the causal chain leading to the patient gaining access to the service in question.

Conclusion

This section has provided an overview of three common proposals in the literature for the regulation of conscientious objection. I have argued that none of these proposals yield a morally adequate solution to the "problem" of conscientious objection. None of the proposals can be construed as an adequate compromise between the interests of conscientious objectors and the interests of patients. On the contrary, blanket bans, conscience tribunals and referral requirements give priority to the interests of patients and the judgements of professional associations where there is a clash between the beliefs of a doctor and the treatment preferences of a patient. In doing so, the aforementioned frameworks fail to give due recognition to conscience as an integral part of human moral psychology and, indeed, an essential feature of the moral and technical rationality of a clinician. In the previous two chapters, I argued that conscience is an essential feature of the moral life of human beings and that it tracks those commitments that an agent cannot violate without transgressing the very conditions of their life and identity (McFall 1987). When a pro-life, devoutly Catholic doctor performs an abortion she does more than commit an act that is contrary to her deeply held beliefs; the doctor jeopardises a life project that defines her existence and provides her with a fundamental source of existential orientation and motivation. She also denies her own considered understanding of reality. The act that she carries out is so alien to her fundamental belief system that she is liable to become alienated from herself. It is hard to conceptualise this kind of moral harm, yet by the same token it is hard to overestimate its seriousness. Indeed, the existential cost of violating one's deepest moral commitments provides us with a strong "prima facie case for accommodation" of conscientious objection in healthcare (Wicclair 2017, 16).

2. Minimising conflict and ensuring access to services

This book has made the case for the protection of conscience rights and the accommodation of conscientious objectors in the healthcare system. I have not, however, engaged extensively with countervailing considerations related to issues of access for patients and the importance of adherence to the moral norms of the medical profession. This is largely because I think the supposed "conflict" between conscientious objection and patient rights/professional authority is illusory. Conscience is central to medicine, and so we should not think of it as coming into conflict with anything. That being said, we can still comment on how one might minimise the supposed "conflict" while keeping in view our fundamental rejection of the idea that conscience is somehow inessential in medical practice. In what follows I will focus on practical solutions within the healthcare system that can help us to meet the interests of the profession and patients while also protecting the rights of conscientious objectors. I will first discuss potential legislative solutions to the problem of conscientious objection. I will then consider the notion of a conscientious objection register as well as a quota system and a system of doctor-patient matching.

Some theorists propose that we should seek legislative solutions to the problem of conscientious objection. That is to say, we should seek to introduce legislation that protects the rights of conscientious objectors or that somehow balances the interests of conscientious objectors with that of patients. Oderberg (2018), for example, offers an extensive discussion of the practicalities of enshrining conscience protections in the laws of a particular jurisdiction. He argues that lawmakers ought to introduce conscientious objection clauses into equality laws rather than introducing specific legislation dealing with conscientious objection in healthcare. Oderberg suggests that such legislation would be more effective in achieving the goal of protecting conscientious objectors; he also appears to believe that it would have more chance of receiving parliamentary support.

Oderberg suggests that any conscience clause integrated into equality legislation ought to be sufficiently broad so as to ensure wide-ranging protections for conscientious objectors. He suggests legislative wording along the following lines:

> [N]o individual, whether through their own agency or the agency of a corporation or other legally recognised body, shall be required to provide, participate in, cooperate with, or refer for, any goods or services of a health-care-related nature contrary to that individual's conscientious beliefs, religious beliefs or moral convictions.
>
> (2018, 122)

Oderberg suggests that the legislative provision may be applied to both government and non-government bodies, as the government ought not to "play favorites" in determining which legal rights ought to be prioritised.

Interestingly, the Australian government recently released draft religious discrimination legislation that sought to provide protection to healthcare practitioners with a religious objection to certain medical procedures. Section 8(6) of the second exposure draft of the *Religious Discrimination Bill 2019* (Cth) stated that

> if a law of a State or Territory allows a health practitioner to conscientiously object to providing a health service because of a religious belief or activity held or engaged in by the health practitioner, a health practitioner conduct rule that is not consistent with that law is not reasonable.

The legislation sought to protect people of faith from rules imposed by healthcare providers or medical bodies that require practitioners to provide (or refer for) particular medical services. While the clause was ultimately removed from the bill, it does provide an illustrative example of what legislative protection for conscientious objectors might look like. The clause in the proposed Australian religious discrimination legislation is not dissimilar from Oderberg's legislative proposal, though its scope is narrowed by its recognition of existing state and territory legislation.

While I am not averse to legislative solutions for regulating conscientious objection, such legislation is not without challenges. For one, it is difficult to devise legislation that adequately balances the rights of conscientious objectors with patients and the medical profession in a manner satisfactory to all stakeholders. It would seem that broad-ranging legislation is doomed to inadequately accommodate the interests of patients and the medical profession on the one hand and the rights of conscientious objectors on the other. Insofar as this is the case, conscience legislation is unlikely to achieve majority support. The law, furthermore, is an instrument that is good for outlining general principles and statutes but not particularly useful in yielding nuanced guidelines for the handling of individual cases. It does not seem particularly amenable to providing nuanced resolutions to individual disputes between conscientious objectors and patients.

One might argue that legislation could be made sufficiently fine-grained so as to provide a system of reconciling the conflicting interests of patients and objecting doctors. Some conscience-based legislation, for example, seeks to give conscience rights to healthcare practitioners while (i) requiring them to provide referrals to patients seeking a service that they will not provide and (ii) requiring them to perform the relevant procedures in emergency situations where the patient's life is at risk. The basic objection, nevertheless, still stands: the task of drafting conscientious objection legislation appears exceedingly difficult given the multifarious situations in which conflicts of conscience might occur. Referral requirements only address one of many potential conflict situations that might arise in clinical practice. The law does not seem to be sufficiently subtle to reconcile the interests of conscientious objectors with those of patients.

A reader might wonder what my attitude is towards existing conscience legislation such as the conscience clauses inherent in U.S. federal healthcare law. U.S. federal law recognises the right of healthcare institutions to refuse to participate in the provision of abortions and voluntary sterilisations. The "Church Amendments" – conscience-based statutes enacted federally in 1973 – state that public funding for religious healthcare facilities should not be conditional on the provision of these services (Bertelsen 2013). The Church Amendments provide broad protection to religiously affiliated hospitals who do wish to provide abortion. One might wonder whether the sceptical analysis of conscience-based legislation advanced earlier applies to the existing conscience-based legislation of this kind.

I have no objection to the Church Amendments in the United States, in part because they were enacted at a time when opposition to conscientious objection was far less pronounced than it is today.[3] In the liberal democracies of our current era, however, it would be much more difficult to achieve bipartisan support for legislation providing broad protection for the rights of conscientious objectors. Rather, attempt at such legislation is unfortunately likely to reignite partisan disputes about abortion or related issues. With this in view, it strikes me that legislative solutions may not be the best approach to resolving disputes between objecting doctors, their patients and the medical profession generally.

In lieu of the broad-ranging legislative regulation of conscientious objection, I would argue that we should focus on practical solutions within the healthcare system that can help us to meet the interests of the profession and patients while also protecting the rights of conscientious objectors. It is appropriate here to consider the possibility of a public register either for *conscientious objectors* or *conscientious providers* (i.e. physicians willing to provide a particular service). We can then consider how quotas for conscientious objectors in the medical profession or a system of doctor-patient matching may help us avoid the key issues of conflict that critics of conscientious objection focus on.

One might argue that the first step in achieving practicable solutions to the conflicts arising from conscientious objection is to introduce a conscientious objection register whereby we can easily identify which doctors are conscientious objectors and which are not. It would be difficult to develop a workable system for regulating conscientious objection if we did not have some reliable means by which we can identify practitioners who are conscientious objectors. A professional register would be one means of determining which practitioners have a conscientious objection to what procedures and which practitioners are willing to perform a full suite of legally sanctioned and safe medical procedures. Specifically, one could argue that we ought to make it a requirement that conscientious objectors declare their conscientious objection to a public body such as a professional college or medical regulator.

One potential challenge, however, would be to avoid the politicisation of the register in such a way that it reflected a negative view of conscientious objection. This is exemplified in the model of a conscientious objection register proposed by Fernandez-Lynch (2008). Fernandez-Lynch suggests that the onus should be on conscientiously objecting physicians to register their objection with a state licensing board, as conscientious objectors "are opting to narrow their portion of the profession's obligation and because it would simply be most efficient" (2008, 145). The registration of one's conscientious objection would give boards

> clear data about the availability of various medical services falling under the profession's obligation, at least as affected by physician conscience, since they could assume that licensees who register no objections are morally willing to provide all services covered by their specialty.
>
> (2008, 145)

Physicians who fail to register their conscientious objection would face appropriate consequences. They would be confronted with:

> "a choice between compliance with the patient's request despite moral objections or forfeiture of conscience clause protection, resulting in some sort of disciplinary and/or liability consequence for refusal."
>
> (2008, 145)

A failure of a conscientious objector to register, in other words, would mean a forfeiture of one's right to conscientious objection.

One problem with Fernandez-Lynch's model is that it assumes that conscientious objectors "are opting to narrow their portion of the profession's obligation" (2008, 145). The reality is that many conscientious objectors would argue that the services to which they object are not part of their professional obligations. Rather, they fall beyond the ambit of what constitutes good medicine. As such, it seems that this justification for placing the onus on conscientious objectors to register their objection seems inadequate. An efficiency justification may provide a more plausible rationale for asking conscientious objectors to register their views. But one would still need to be careful about construing this as a requirement justified by the burden that conscientious objection places on patients and the healthcare system.

A deeper problem with a conscientious objection register is that it is profoundly offensive to require citizens in a democratic state to register their intention to exercise fundamental freedoms. There are inoffensive reasons to have a register for sex offenders and gun and car owners, but not those wishing to exercise freedom of expression (or of certain kinds of expression). It would be wrong to require doctors to make an official declaration about their intention to practise medicine in accord with their conscience (presuming that their actions fall within the criteria of reasonableness outlined in the previous chapter). Doctors should be allowed to practise in the manner they deem appropriate provided that they are not violating professional guidelines or falling afoul of basic professional standards. There is nothing about this that is contrary to one's professional duties.

There is also a practical dimension to this concern arising from the fact that conscience is integral to medical practice. It is often the case that a physician may object to procedure X in certain circumstances but not in others. How would a doctor express this in a declaration to medical regulators? Would the doctor be required to write a detailed account of the multifarious situations that might lead them to exercise their right to conscientious non-participation? Or should we rather respect the discretion of medical practitioners? It is a mistake to assume that the question "Will you provide?" always has a yes-or-no answer. It may often be "it depends". As such, a conscientious objection register may not be a workable solution to the problem of ensuring access.

Rather, it may be the case that the most appropriate solution is to establish a register of *conscientious providers*. That is to say, we should establish a register of practitioners who are categorically willing to provide a particular service and are morally committed to ensuring that the service is readily available to patients. In the case of euthanasia, for example, we could have a register of practitioners who are trained and ready to provide euthanasia to patients and who are appropriately located (or willing to travel) to ensure that such services are accessible. Physicians could be encouraged to come forward and register their willingness to provide particular services – be it euthanasia or another contentious service – where there is a genuine, evidence-based concern about the impact that conscientious objection may have on service provision.

A register of *conscientious providers* appears to avoid the objections raised earlier. Such a register would not have the same risk of politicisation as a conscientious objection register as it would not be based on an assumption that the practitioners who make up the register are somehow neglecting their professional duties. Nor could it be interpreted as a register that requires people to indicate their intention to exercise fundamental human rights. On the contrary, the register would be based on an appeal by the state for practitioners to come forward and agree to provide a service that is sanctioned by the law. If anything, it would seem that there may be professional advantages for clinicians to register their intention to provide services that are sanctioned in law and endorsed by the state.

A register of conscientious providers may also be more practicable than a register of conscientious objectors. Assuming that conscientious providers are very willing and able to provide a service to whosoever requests that service as per the circumscriptions of the law, then there would be less of a concern about imposing unworkable requirements on physicians. The register could ask, "Will you provide this service?" as it is precisely directed at clinicians who have no moral reservations about the service in question and deem the service to be morally important to society. The issue, if anything, would be finding a sufficient number of practitioners who fall into this category of full willingness to provide services. If, indeed, we could not find a sufficient number of practitioners who would sign up to the register, we would need to consider whether the issue lay with doctors or whether in fact the issue was to be found in the morality of the procedure in question.

Health authorities might also advise objectors to notify patients and employers of their position in advance once it becomes clear that a conflict may arise. This would be aimed at avoiding and minimising conflict and facilitating alternative access to services. In an institutional setting this would, in practice, result in an institutional register of objectors, but this kind of arrangement would be more limited and specifically tailored to practical needs. Objecting physicians may find this significantly less objectionable or offensive.

What if these measures failed to ensure adequate access to services? In this situation, it would seem that it would be necessary to determine an alternative means by which we could reconcile the interests of patients seeking legal medical services and the interests of the conscientious objectors who refuse to provide certain procedures. Two options proposed in the literature that I believe are worthy of exploration are (i) quotas for conscientious objectors and (ii) a system of doctor-patient matching based on patient preferences and physician beliefs.

A quota system would require that we establish quotas within relevant medical specialities for objecting physicians and non-objecting physicians. The aim of this system would be to ensure that there are a sufficient number of physicians available within a particular speciality to provide all services desired by patients. A quota system would also ensure that objecting physicians had at least some assurance that they would be eligible for a position within the profession in question. The quota system, in other words, should not focus on patient interests to the exclusion of the rights of objecting doctors. On the contrary, it should be impartial with respect to the conflicting rights at play. With this in view, Rodger and Blackshaw (2021) have suggested that quotas in medicine might in some cases be 50/50 with respect to conscientiously objecting physicians and non-objecting physicians (though this would really depend on the number of applicants who were conscientious objectors, and this would be a maximum with no minimal requirement). Alternatively, we might set the quota based on the minimum number of new physicians estimated to be needed to provide services to which conscientious objection is common.

A quota system could be introduced for all physicians who are already practising medicine. That is to say, medical authorities could place restrictions on (or even revoke the license of) a certain number of objecting medical practitioners. If the number of objecting practitioners was too high, medical authorities could randomly select an appropriate number of these practitioners to be redeployed according to the quota. Alternatively, a certain number of conscientious objectors could be admitted to practise in a particular geographic area while several non-objecting physicians could be redeployed. This will be easier or more challenging depending on the kind of healthcare system in place.

Yet this approach would be incredibly draconian and unfair to physicians who are already working and who joined the profession believing that their job would be under threat because they had a conscientious objection (or, alternatively, because they did not have an objection). As such, one might consider whether quotas ought to come into play at the time at which physicians seek admission to a particular medical college. Applicants to the college could be informed of the policy and be required to declare their position vis-à-vis particular services that members of the college are likely to be asked to provide. If an applicant is unwilling to provide these services, they can still proceed with their application to the college, though they would need to be informed that their chances of succeeding in their application are indexed to the quota of conscientious objectors for that particular year.

Rodger and Blackshaw (2021) argue that a quota system would allow us to deal with two opposite problems that arise in relation to conscientious objection. First, a quota would allow us to address the problem of a lack of access to services like abortion that one finds in Italy and other socially conservative nations. Quotas would ensure that a sufficient number of willing medical professionals are available to provide abortion services in any one region of the country. Second, quotas would ensure that conscientiously objecting medical professionals are not unfairly barred from any one medical speciality. Quotas would ensure, for example, that religious doctors with an objection to abortion are not barred from admission to medical specialities such as obstetrics and gynaecology in liberal democratic nations like Canada (Schuklenk and Smalling 2017) or the United Kingdom (Savulescu 2006).

Whatever the apparent merits of quotas, I would be very cautious about the adoption of a quota system for regulating conscientious objection in the medical profession. For one, it is not entirely clear how we ought to go about determining what proportion of objecting doctors ought to be allowed into particular medical specialties. A balance would need to be struck between not discriminating against conscientious objectors and ensuring that a maximum number of medical students are able to be recruited. Quotas could become an artificial construct that are simply a band-aid solution to more fundamental issues at the heart of the conscientious objection debate. It is fundamentally pragmatic (or ambitious in countries that do not allow conscientious objection). Quotas may not even provide any benefits for patients seeking medical services. It is not entirely clear that high rates of conscientious objection directly correlate with issues of a lack of access to particular medical services. Admittedly, Rodger and Blackshaw deal with this objection by reviewing the empirical literature on conscientious objection and conclude that

> there is evidence for a link between conscientious objection and compromised access to abortion services, but it is limited to areas where levels of conscientious objection are very high.
>
> (2021, 158)

Government support for medical services also plays a significant role in determining what patients can access. One would need to ascertain that a quota system would indeed effectively address the challenges attended to access to medical services in a particular region.

A quota system is also offensive and inappropriate if indeed conscience is integral to medicine, as I have argued in the early chapters of this book. If conscience is integral to medicine then quotas start to look like restrictions on the number of doctors in the profession who will practise medicine in an authentic way. We might inadvertently limit the number of physicians who genuinely use their conscience when discerning what to do in particular situations. Rather, we could be fostering a culture of regimentation in medicine whereby the state limits the number of conscientious medical practitioners and instead focuses on ensuring that enough practitioner-apparatchiks are available to implement its legal mandates concerning contentious socio-clinical services (Gamble and Pruski 2019).

Finally, many "conscientious objectors" do not even need to make decisions which conflict with professional guidelines. Their conscientious objection never takes the form of a conflict because they never have to deal with the kinds of procedures to which they might have an objection (consider, for example, a radiologist who has an objection to abortion). Quotas – be they introduced at medical school or at some later point in one's professional development – would falsely inflate the role of conscientious objectors with regard to obstructing access to healthcare. Quotas are perhaps underpinned by a mistaken assumption that all conscientious objectors will necessarily obstruct access to morally contentious services in some way.

To be clear, I am not entirely averse to the idea of seeking some sort of balance between conscientious objection and access to services in a particular medical speciality. I also commend Rodger and Blackshaw (2021) for attempting to find a practicable solution to the ideological impasse on the regulation of conscientious objection. I am, however, unconvinced that the introduction of quotas would be the most effective way to realise this goal. Quotas could end up being an artificial fix that failed to achieve the goal of "keeping the peace" between conscientious objectors, the medical profession in general and patients. Rather, they could generate ire against the government for placing restrictions on the expression of practitioner values, whatever they may be. It would be likely that at least one (if not all) of the stakeholders involved would be unhappy with the solution.

Rodger and Blackshaw have acknowledged that there is a long way between proposing a quota framework and actually implementing a quota system that is feasible and useful. They suggest that it would be most useful initially to introduce conscientious objection via a quota into a jurisdiction that currently does not allow it. This process would give a lot of useful data on effects and usefulness of quotas. Importantly, if quotas were introduced at a fairly low level and in fairly tightly circumscribed circumstances, then they would be unlikely to affect abortion access or access to other social contentious medical practices.

An alternative option to quotas would be to introduce a doctor-patient matching system into the medical profession. One specific proposal in the literature is that we should allow practitioners to avoid workplaces where their values are likely to be compromised. Indeed, Fernandez-Lynch (2008) has argued that doctor-patient matching on the basis of personal moral values would eliminate, or at least minimise, many conflicts of conscience. She suggests that state licensing boards ought to facilitate this goal. Many institutions, Fernandez-Lynch contends – such as pharmacies, hospitals and medical schools – would not be well suited for the task of doctor-patient matching. Licensing boards, however, are well placed for balancing the interests of doctors and patients by ensuring a sufficient number of willing physicians are available such that no physician's refusal leaves a patient entirely without access to desired medical services.

Fernandez-Lynch (2008) goes to some length to consider the practical implications of a system of doctor-patient matching for conscientious objection. She outlines a system for determining which conscientious objections ought to fall within the ambit of state protection. She considers how hospitals and healthcare providers might handle the transition of patients from an objecting to a non-objecting clinician. She also provides a detailed overview of how we might ensure that a sufficient number of clinicians are available in particular geographic areas to ensure ease of access to services for patients. She notes several challenges in determining what is sufficiently "easy" access to service and in what cases conscientious objection can be said to be the primary issue.

Fernandez-Lynch (2008) suggests that a system of doctor-patient matching could be implemented in concert with several other measures to ensure adequate access to services for patients. One such measure would be incentives for doctors who were willing to provide particular kinds of medical services. Doctors could be offered financial incentives, for example, if they were willing to provide services that were in demand in particular areas but that are also difficult to access on account of high rates of conscientious objection (Fernandez-Lynch 2008, 188). Another measure might be to offer special visas to appropriately qualified physicians from other nations under the proviso that they would practise in particular geographical areas and provide particular services (Fernandez-Lynch 2008, 184–185). The author, however, suggests that this approach should be used as a last resort so as to avoid a brain drain in developing countries. Fernandez-Lynch also acknowledges that there may be some hard cases where limited restrictions on conscientious objection are deemed appropriate (for example, where a doctor is the only physician in a town, and it is not feasible for patients to travel to other towns to access services that the doctor is competent to provide but to which they nevertheless have a moral objection) (Fernandez-Lynch 2008, 198–199).

Fernandez-Lynch is to be commended for her attempt to find a practicable solution to what has been a long-standing problem with medical practice. Her solution, furthermore, is certainly not one to be trivially dismissed. Rather, in the notion of doctor-patient matching one finds the basis of what might just be the most promising way to resolve ongoing tensions over the exercise of conscience in healthcare. Unlike quotas, a system of doctor-patient matching would not place limits on medical students who hold particular values and who nevertheless wish to train as doctors and enter particular medical specialties. It also seems that a fine-grained system of matching could do a much better job of ensuring appropriate levels of access to services for patients.

There are, however, significant issues with the author's proposed system that would require a major reworking of the model of a doctor-patient matching system. One problem raised by E.L. Bedford (2018) is that the doctor-patient matching system could easily lapse into a system of tight restrictions on the practice of conscientiously objecting doctors. He writes that Fernandez-Lynch's model could

> limit the freedom of physicians to choose where they live and practice. Currently, this is the choice of the physician based on essentially free market principles. This solution would add a layer of bureaucratic centralized planning that would seem oppressive for a profession that is already among the most regulated.
>
> (2018, 242)

Indeed, it is not entirely clear how far Fernandez-Lynch intends to take her system. Would it, for example, create geographical locations where it is very difficult for conscientious objectors to find employment? And what might happen to objecting practitioners if the demographics of their current place of work change such that there is greater need for access to controversial medical services?

Bedford argues that any "solution" to the problem of conscientious objection needs to include reference to institutions as intermediaries between the individual and the state. He writes:

> [A] comprehensive approach to the CO debate must address the social, mediating space between the individual and the state, the realm of the institution.
>
> (2018, 242)

Institutions are an ineradicable feature of societies in general and healthcare systems in particular. It behoves us to consider what role institutions might play in ensuring not only that patients have access to the services they desire but also that institutions exist where doctors with a conscientious objection can practise in good conscience (and patients who share the views of objecting physicians can receive care in an environment friendly to such views).

The issue remains, however, that a system of doctor-patient matching could relegate conscientiously objecting physicians to particular institutions that are for various reasons unideal places of work. Many religious hospitals, for example – where conscientious objectors might be able to practise in accord with their beliefs – are private institutions and do not have the same patient flow and access to cutting-edge technologies and treatment modalities as public institutions. Relegation of conscientious objectors to private hospitals may compromise their training and impose an inadvertent "conscientious apartheid" in medical training opportunities.

This may present yet another reason why an optional and searchable database of doctors with no conscientious objection should be devised. Patients could be directed to search this database to find an appropriate practitioner. This would protect the privacy of conscientiously objecting doctors, prevent politicisation and also optimise patient access to care.

These criticisms notwithstanding, one attractive feature of Fernandez-Lynch's model is that it does not place the onus on either patients or doctors to deal with the tensions created by conscientious objection. If any organisation were to be put in charge of guaranteeing appropriate doctor-patient matching, it seems it should be a governmental body. One could argue that governments have the responsibility to ensure that legislation is implemented in a manner that does not restrict any citizen's liberty. In the case of conscientious objection, governments have obligations to ensure that conscientious objectors can carry out their work appropriately even where this means that the government must create alternative access options for patients. That is to say, governments ought to take responsibility for ensuring that practitioners are available to provide relevant medical services to patients – this should not be seen as a responsibility of medical practitioners themselves.

As I stated at the beginning of the chapter, my aim is not to provide a comprehensive overview of how conscientious objection ought to be regulated in practice. Such a task is beyond the scope of this book. I do, however, believe that some variant of a doctor-patient matching system – perhaps based on a database of *conscientious providers* – is a more promising and practicable option than other proposals such as broad-reaching legislation or quotas.

Conclusion

In this chapter I have discussed the regulation of conscientious objection in healthcare practice and have discussed policies whereby we might ensure that the conscience rights of healthcare practitioners are respected. In Section 1, I discussed recent suggestions by critics of conscientious protections about how we should regulate the practice of conscientious objection in healthcare. I argued against blanket bans on conscientious objection, as well as criticising proposals in favour of conscience tribunals and referral requirements for practitioners who conscientiously object. In Section 2, I explored positive proposals for how conscience rights might be respected. I argued that legislative solutions may be unlikely to placate the different stakeholders involved in the healthcare system. A public register of practitioners' willingness to provide particular services, as well as a system of doctor-patient matching, may constitute a viable option for ensuring that neither doctors' nor patients' preferences are unnecessarily affected. Our discussion would not be complete, however, without a consideration of the ethics of institutional conscientious objection. It is to this topic that we now turn.

Notes

1   I am here presuming, for argument's sake, that there is a conflict between physicians' rights and patients' access to services. In reality, however, conscience is integral to medical practice and so ought not to be seen as the source of the problem. The problem, if indeed there is one, lies with medical authorities' failure to ensure that there are a

sufficient number of clinicians available who are willing to perform the services in question. I discuss this in Section 3 of this chapter.

2 See Carter Snead. *What It Means to Be Human: The Case for the Body in Public Bioethics.* Cambridge: Harvard University Press, 2020.

3 If I were to identify a shortcoming of this legislation, it would be the focus on religious objections to abortions and voluntary sterilisations rather than ethical objections in general. A healthcare institution may have an objection to these procedures even if it is not religious.

References

Bedford, E.L. "Book review: Conflicts of conscience in healthcare: An institutional compromise". *The Linacre Quarterly* 86;2–3 (2018): 240–242.

Bertelsen, S. "Conscientious objection of health care providers: Lessons from the experience of the United States". *Notre Dame Journal of International & Comparative Law* 3;1 (2013): 122–148.

Card, R.F. "Conscientious objection, emergency contraception, and public policy". *Journal of Medicine and Philosophy* 36;1 (2011): 53–68.

Card, R.F. "In defence of medical tribunals and the reasonability standard for conscientious objection in medicine". *Journal of Medical Ethics* 42 (2016): 73–75.

Card, R.F. "Reasons, reasonability and establishing conscientious objector status in medicine". *Journal of Medical Ethics* 43 (2017): 222–225.

Charo, Alta. "The celestial fire of conscience – refusing to deliver medical care". *The Journal of Medical Ethics* 352;24 (2005): 2471–2473.

Clarke, S. "Conscientious objection in healthcare, referral, and the military analogy". *Journal of Medical Ethics* 43 (2017a): 218–221.

Clarke, S. "Two concepts of conscience and their implications for conscience-based refusal in healthcare". *Journal of Medical Ethics* 26 (2017b): 97–108.

College of Physicians and Surgeons of Ontario. *News Release* 6th March 2015. Available from www.cpso.on.ca.

Cowley, C. "Conscientious objection in healthcare and the duty to refer". *Journal of Medical Ethics* 43 (2017): 207–212.

Curlin, Farr, and Tollefsen, Christopher. *The Way of Medicine: Ethics and the Healing Professions.* South Bend: University of Notre Dame Press, 2021.

Eberl, Jason. "Conscientious objection in health care". *Theoretical Medicine and Bioethics* 40;6 (2019): 483–486.

Fernandez-Lynch, Holly. *Conflicts of Conscience in Health Care: An Institutional Compromise.* Cambridge, MA: MIT Press, 2008.

Gamble, Nathan, and Pruski, Michal. "Medical acts and conscientious objection: What can a physician be compelled to do?". *The New Bioethics* 25 (2019): 262–282.

Hughes, Jonathan. "Conscientious objection in healthcare: Why tribunals might be the answer". *Journal of Medical Ethics* 43 (2017): 213–217.

Keogh, Louise, Gillam, Lynn, Bismarck, Marie *et al.* "Conscientious objection to abortion, the law and its implementation in Victoria, Australia: Perspectives of abortion service providers". *BMC Medical Ethics* 20;11 (2019): 11.

Kessler, Jeremy. "A war for liberty: On the law of conscientious objection". In Michael Geyer and Adam Tooze (eds.). *The Cambridge History of the Second World War Vol. 3: Total War: Economy, Society and Culture.* London: Cambridge University Press, 2015: 447–474.

McDermott, James. *British Military Service Tribunals, 1916–1918*. Manchester University Press, 2011.

McFall, Lynn. "Integrity". *Ethics* 98;1 (1987): 5–20.

McLeod, Carolyn. *Conscience in Reproductive Health Care: Prioritizing Patient Interests*. London: Oxford University Press, 2020.

Oderberg, David. *Opting Out: Conscience and Cooperation in a Pluralist Society*. London: Institute for Economic Affairs, 2018.

Rodger, Daniel, and Blackshaw, Bruce. "Quotas: Enabling conscientious objection to coexist with abortion access". *Health Care Analysis* 29 (2021): 154–169.

Savulescu, Julian. "Conscientious objection in medicine". *British Medical Journal* 332 (2006): 294–297.

Savulescu, Julian, and Schuklenk, Udo. "Doctors have no right to refuse medical assistance in dying, abortion or contraception". *Bioethics* 31;3 (2017): 162–170.

Schuklenk, Udo, and Smalling, Ricardo. "Why medical professionals have no moral claim to conscientious objection accommodation in liberal democracies". *Journal of Medical Ethics* 43 (2017): 234–240.

Stahl, Ronit, and Emanuel, Ezekiel. "Physicians not conscripts; conscientious objection in healthcare". *The New England Journal of Medicine* 376;14 (2017): 1380–1385.

Sulmasy, Daniel. "Tolerance, professional judgement, and the discretionary space of the physician". *Cambridge Quarterly of Healthcare Ethics* 21;6 (2017): 18–31.

Symons, Xavier. "Pellegrino, MacIntyre, and the internal morality of clinical medicine". *Theoretical Medicine and Bioethics* 40;3 (2019): 243–251.

Trigg, R. "Conscientious objection and 'effective referral'". *Cambridge Quarterly of Healthcare Ethics* 26 (2017): 32–43.

Wicclair, M. "Managing conscientious objection in health care institutions". *HEC Forum* 26 (2014): 267–283.

Wicclair, M. "Conscientious objection in healthcare and moral integrity". *Cambridge Quarterly of Healthcare Ethics* 26;1 (2017): 7–17.

6 The permissibility of institutional conscientious objection

Introduction

In this chapter, I will explore whether institutions have a conscience and whether this matters for the permissibility of conscientious objection. I will focus in particular on the costliness of violating deeply held beliefs and will consider what relevance this notion might have for our understanding of the ethics of institutional conscientious objection. I have argued that conscience is a notion that is essential to understanding the phenomenon of conscientious objection, such that one would be forgiven for thinking that entities that lack a conscience are not deserving of conscience rights. I will, however, argue against this assumption. Even if institutions do not have a conscience, there is still good moral justification for granting them what I call *conscience rights** (or rights analogous to conscience rights for individuals). I will argue that an institution's mission and values are analogous to the considered and deeply held beliefs that conscience monitors. Just as we respect the deeply held beliefs of individuals, so too should we respect the right to conscientious objection of institutions.

This chapter is partly motivated by two very different claims made in the bioethics literature. The first is the claim that institutions have consciences and that this makes them deserving of the right to institutional conscientious objection. Sulmasy (2008, 144) writes that "health care institutions have consciences, at least by a strong analogy if not also in fact", whereas Bedford (2016, 265) writes that "institutional conscience stands as an integral and inextricable dimension of every human institution". The second, contrasting claim in the literature is the view that institutions do not have consciences and therefore are not deserving of conscience protections. Spencer Durland, for example, writes that institutions do not have a psychology or free will and therefore should not be afforded conscience rights*. He argues that

> a hospital is not a person; it is a physical structure within which providers give medical care. It does not perform procedures or counsel patients. It does not take lunch hours or vacations. And it does not have a conscience.
>
> (2011, 1659)

DOI: 10.4324/9781003247623-6

Duland goes on to argue that appeals to institutional conscience are "indefensible" and that "the notion of institutional conscience must simply be dropped from conscience legislation" (2011, 1659).

Pace Sulmasy and Bedford, I will argue that institutions *do not* have consciences. There is no sense in which institutions possess a conscience akin to individual moral agents. It is only individual moral agents who have a capacity for conscious moral reflection that is characteristic of the action of conscience. Pace Durland, however, I still believe that institutions deserve to have their liberties protected. I will present arguments in favour of conscience rights* that do not depend on the existence of institutional conscience for their success. Rather, these arguments are concerned with the protection of individual conscience and the preservation of institutional integrity.

In Section 1, I offer a brief discussion of the metaphysics of institutions. In Section 2, I discuss whether institutions have a conscience. I argue that institutions lack consciousness, and are also not subject to the emotional sanction of conscience, and so cannot be said to have a conscience. In Section 3, I consider whether the question of conscience matters to the permissibility of institutional conscientious objection. I argue that there are independent reasons for respecting the autonomy and core beliefs of institutions. I argue that institutional liberty is important for the protection of individual conscience. That is to say, institutional liberty is important if we are to respect an individual agent's right to conscientious objection. I also argue that institutional integrity is important for the good of both institutions in themselves and society at large.

1. What is an institution?

It is apposite to begin this chapter with a rough definition of the term "institution".[1] Admittedly, "institution" is a word that is used fairly loosely in everyday discourse, and it can refer to various kinds of social entities. Viewed from one perspective, institutions might be thought to be social structures or practices that persist over a long period of time. One example might be the Crown of England – a monarchical governmental structure that has arguably persisted from sometime in the 9th century (around the time of Egbert) through to Elizabeth II (Rust 2019, 13). Alternatively, we might think of institutions as important and influential organisations within a given society. Some examples of influential social institutions include financial institutions, like the U.S. Federal Reserve, or educational institutions, like the University of Oxford. There are also community institutions that help sustain the social fabric of societies, like government or charitable institutions that are responsible for the provision of social services and healthcare.

It is instructive for our purposes to consider the basic characteristics of institutions so as to come to a working definition of this type of social entity. First, we can say that institutions are greater than the sum of the individual moral agents which compose them. Many institutions have existed for several decades or even multiple centuries or millennia, and, as such, they must by definition transcend any particular individual or set of individual members. If the English Crown were defined by a particular person, then it would have ceased to exist when that person ceased to exist. Second, institutions are not necessarily limited to particular physical locations, though often they are centred on a particular physical site or a series of sites. If we were to claim that institutions have a fixed physical location or embodiment, then we would be unable to explain how many institutions perdure even when their physical location changes over time. The fact that institutions are not defined by a particular physical location or even a particular historical period means that we need to look elsewhere to find a means of defining what institutions are.

In this chapter, I will be focusing in particular on *healthcare institutions*. I want to suggest that a very important part of this kind of institution is the core commitments that define it and, related to this, the history, heritage and practices associated with the institution. In the end, the core ideals and aims of institutions are what appear to unite the various people and the various physical manifestations that make up an institution over the course of time. The shared mission and goals of members of institutions provide a bond that brings unity to the very varied circumstances in which individual members of the institution find themselves. This consideration, as we shall see, lends support to the idea that the protection of institutional ideals is of significant moral importance and that we should not be dismissive of appeals to institutional integrity in the context of debates about conscientious objection.

A critic might try to resist this emphasis on an institution's values and heritage. Yet we need some criterion for determining who is a member of an institution, and it is unclear whether there are any other features of healthcare institutions that could be said to unite every individual member. Consider, for example, St Vincent's Hospital in Sydney, Australia – a healthcare institution that has existed since the mid-1800s. The members of the institution who were active in its early history – Irish Sisters of Charity trained in nursing who migrated to Australia for the purposes of providing healthcare to the poor and disadvantaged – would have lived and worked in very different circumstances to employees of the organisation today. There seems to be very little that unites the past and present members of the organisation other than a shared historical narrative and a series of core commitments that have endured throughout the organisation's history. The organisation's ethos of care, for example, might be a unifying feature in the disparate experiences of its employees over the years. We should, therefore, acknowledge that the philosophy of care of an institution as well as its history and heritage are very important parts of its identity. Indeed, other aspects of these institutions, such as their current physical location and current staff population, are contingent features of the organisation and are arguably not as important to defining the institution as its mission, aims and heritage. An institution's mission, aims and heritage are central to its identity.

To be clear, I am not claiming that institutions will cease to exist if they change one or other aspect of their mission or values. Certainly there are other aspects of an institution – such as its physical location, its status in the eyes of the law and its social role that plausibly plays some role in constituting its identity. But institutional values are certainly a very important part of identity, and there is a sense in which the identity of an institution can fracture when it changes its values. We will return to this idea in the final sections of this thesis.

2. Do institutions have a conscience?

In this section, I will consider whether institutions have consciences. It is my contention that institutions *do not* have a conscience – at least not in the sense defined in this book – as they lack consciousness and do not experience emotions. The discussion has three subsections. In the subsection named "The nature of conscience" I offer a brief account of the nature of conscience that draws upon the discussion in Chapter 3. I try to stay at a sufficient level of generality to avoid simply presuming that non-human entities are unable to have a conscience. In the subsection titled " Institutions, conscience and consciousness", I will consider whether institutions are conscious entities (something I take to be a sine qua non for the possession of a conscience). In the subsection titled " Institutions and the emotional sanction of conscience", I will consider whether institutions are subject to the emotional sanction of conscience.

The nature of conscience

In this section I will provide a minimal account of conscience drawing upon the discussion in Chapter 3. It should suffice to outline some basic criteria that characterise conscience qua a principle of moral awareness and a monitor of deeply held beliefs. Specifically, I will rely on three individually necessary and jointly sufficient criteria: the possession of deeply held moral beliefs, the presence of a mechanism that monitors the implementation of these deeply held moral beliefs, and the costliness of going against one's deep beliefs and ignoring the mechanism responsible for monitoring psychological integrity.

First, an entity must have deeply held moral beliefs. By this I am referring to beliefs that are long-standing and firmly held and that to some extent reflect the basic values of a person. Indeed, the sorts of beliefs that philosophers see as relevant to conscience are beliefs that are so central to our outlook on the world that they to some extent define who we are (Sulmasy 2008; Velleman 2009; Lyons 2009; McLeod 2020). Viewed from a developmental perspective, these beliefs often take the form of basic moral maxims that one learnt in childhood or adolescence and that have been mentally sifted and reinforced in adulthood (Lyons 2009, 492). Our views on the metaphysics and value of human life, for example, might be candidates for deep beliefs, depending on the force with which we hold these convictions. Similarly, one's basic understanding of one's familial duties and one's obligations to one's close friends might form part of the contents of conscience. Alternatively, we might think of the ground projects that characterise and give purpose to a mature agent's life. We might think of the professional responsibilities of an agent, as well as their non-professional life goals. Alternatively, we might think of the religious commitments that are central to the sense of purpose and meaning of agent.

The reader may wonder whether "depth" is a measure of how strongly one's beliefs are held or whether it is rather a measure of their "centrality" (i.e. how these beliefs are important to one's self-conception and how they are connected to other self-identifying beliefs that an individual holds). I would argue that "depth" is a measure of *both* the strength with which beliefs are held *and* their centrality in the identity of an agent. Indeed, I would argue that the reason why beliefs are said to be strongly held and hard to revise is that they are central to an agent's sense of identity. This is not to deny that it is sometimes important to "retool" conscience when one has for many years fostered prejudicial or self-degrading beliefs such that they have become part of one's identity (McLeod 2020). Yet this process of "retooling" would presumably be quite difficult and demanding for an agent, for the beliefs we are talking about here are the kind of beliefs that shape one's understanding of the world and one's self. They are entrenched in one's psyche, and one would need to rethink one's whole self-conception in the process of revising deeply held beliefs.

Second, an entity must have a mechanism for overseeing the implementation of their deeply held beliefs into practice. This is a common function that philosophers have historically attributed to conscience. Aquinas described conscience as the faculty responsible for applying general moral beliefs to real-world cases (Hoffmann 2011), whereas Kant described conscience as an "inner court" that monitored whether we have acted in accord with the dictates of practical reason (Wood 2008). The basic idea here is that conscience functions as a monitor of the coherence between an agent's deeply held beliefs and commitments (as per the preceding discussion) and their practical actions. It monitors the extent to which one's actions are consonant with those beliefs that are so central to our outlook on the world that they to some extent define who we are. Where we fail to act in accord with our basic, self-identifying beliefs and commitments, conscience censures us and induces feelings of remorse and regret as well as a desire to re-establish harmony between our deeply held beliefs and our practical actions.

Third, it must be costly for an agent to act contrary to their deeply held beliefs. That is to say, it should cost someone to go against their conscience. It is part of our common understanding of conscience that it expresses itself in terms of guilt and shame – emotions that are associated with feelings of discomfort and unease (Cottingham 2009, 733). Furthermore, conscience has substance to it only insofar as it's difficult or costly to override. Where it is the case that someone could disobey their conscience without consequence, then the idea of conscience would seem to have no real relevance to one's moral life. Conscience would be a mute instrument that had no authority over our moral activity. Typically, the force of conscience comes in the form of an awareness of wrongdoing, a fracturing of the self and negative emotions that one experiences where one disobeys one's conscience. Indeed, many commentators describe conscience as having both cognitive and affective dimensions. As I argued in Chapter 3, moral emotions are more a way in which conscience makes an agent aware of its operations and exerts influence on an agent. That is, conscience manifests itself not just at the level of thought but also of emotion (Childress 1979, 322; Sulmasy 2008, 138; Lyons 2009, 493). For the purposes of this chapter, I will take the emotional sanction of conscience to be a characteristic of the costliness of violating conscience.

A critic might want to resist the idea that emotions are an integral part of the costliness of violating conscience. I did, after all, argue that the fracturing of the self is the most serious form of moral harm that one sustains when one violates one's conscience. Yet the following two hypothetical scenarios illustrate the importance of the emotions in the costliness of not acting in accord with one's basic beliefs.

Scenario #1: robot

Imagine a small robotic device that moves around an area the size of a table top. Suppose that scattered across this area are several cylindrical objects, some upright, some on their sides. The device scans the area with its bug-like eyes, then moves about and, using its prosthetic limbs, puts any cylinders lying on their side into an upright position. It remains on alert after all the cylinders are upright and responds to any cylinder falling over by restoring it to its old position. Yet the scientist who created the robot decides to place cylinders in the area that are unstable and tip over whenever they are placed in an upright position. As a result, the robot is unable to fulfil its function.[2]

Scenario #2: psychopathic doctor

Psychopaths have a cold and cognitive understanding of morality (as a social practice, say), but they are not moved by moral reasons. Indeed, they often exhibit a form of moral incompetence such that they are inattentive to the moral permissibility or impermissibility of their actions. Consider a doctor who is a high-functioning psychopath and who has nevertheless accepted a moral code according to which abortion is immoral. One day, this doctor is asked to perform a therapeutic abortion. The doctor recognises that this action goes against her moral code, but she nevertheless obliges her superiors and carries out the procedure. She does not experience any negative emotions or feelings of cognitive dissonance when carrying out the procedure.

The point of these two case studies is to illustrate the importance of the emotions in characterising the sanction of conscience. It is implausible to impute a conscience to the robot or the psychopath, as neither experiences the emotional costliness of violating conscience.

In the case of the robot, it seems a stretch to say that it experiences something analogous to the pangs of conscience when it fails to enact those things which by design it is intended to achieve. One might say that the robot has beliefs, though even this is controversial. It certainly has algorithms in its programming, and it behaves in line with these algorithms. It may have a way of putting into place its "beliefs" by virtue of some machine-learning programme. It believes that the cylinders should be placed upright, and it seeks to bring this about. But even if we ascribe beliefs to the robot, would we say it has a conscience? And would we say it is harmed when it is impeded in putting its beliefs into practice? The robot does not experience the negative emotions that would typically accompany restrictions on conscience. When the unstable cylinders are placed in the area, the robot does not experience psychological distress or emotional turmoil. It seems a stretch, therefore, to say that it is costly for the robot to be impeded in fulfilling its role. The robot is not psychologically harmed when it is subject to restrictions.

We can also consider the case of the psychopathic doctor. Once again, we can ask whether it is appropriate to say that the doctor experiences the emotional sanction of conscience. The answer is "no". In this scenario, the doctor is told to perform a therapeutic abortion. She obliges her superiors and performs the operation. The doctor clearly recognises that her actions conflict with her moral code, but she performs the procedure nonetheless. In this case, the doctor does not experience the emotional sanction of conscience, despite going against her deeply held beliefs. On account of her psychopathy, the doctor does not have a proper psychological awareness of the moral consequences of her actions. Plausibly, then, it is not costly (at least, not in an emotional sense) for this doctor to act contrary to their deeply held beliefs.

By way of clarification, I am not attempting to reduce the sanction of conscience to the moral emotions of guilt and shame. I argued against this point of view in Chapter 3. We should first remember that the sanction of conscience can also take the form of experiences of emotional numbness and a sense of depersonalisation (whereby an agent becomes existentially disengaged from their own life and actions). Second, violations of conscience lead to a fracturing of the self. By a fracturing of the self, I have in mind something deeper than mere psychological harm. I have in mind the kind of harm to a person's moral identity that comes about when an agent acts contrary to his or her deeply-held beliefs. This is precisely the sort of harm that I take to be most characteristic of violations of conscience and most worthy of our attention and concern. We should be careful about caricaturing conscience as consisting solely of "pangs" and "prods". Even still, I *would* argue that experiences like depersonalisation and emotional numbness are directly related to the affective capacities of human beings. Emotional numbness, for example, stems from among other things an incapacity to empathise with others, and this I take to be a form of affective dysfunction in an agent (Vujosevic 2015; Roberts 2019). As such, even these alternative sanctions of conscience have an essentially affective character.[3]

In summary, it seems that there is an essential connection between having a conscience and having the capacity to experience the emotional sanction of conscience when one has violated one's deeply held beliefs. In the scenarios just presented, we intuitively would say that the robot and the psychopath lack a conscience on account of the absence of the action of conscience when they violate their deeply held beliefs.

The question that we are considering is whether institutions have consciences. We should consider, then, whether institutions meet the minimum criteria that we take to signify the existence of conscience. In the remainder of Section 2, I will discuss two reasons why I think we should not attribute the property of having a conscience to institutions. First, to be the bearer of deep beliefs – which I take to be part of the subject matter of conscience – you need to have *consciousness*, and institutions are not conscious entities. Second, for someone to be subject to correction by their conscience, they need to be capable of experiencing some sort of emotional reproof, yet this does not seem to be the case with institutions. I argue that these two considerations give us good reason to refrain from attributing a conscience to institutions.

I will begin with a discussion of consciousness and a consideration of why it is implausible to attribute consciousness to institutions. I will then turn to a consideration of the emotional sanction that conscience imposes and will argue that this is absent in the case of institutions.

Institutions, conscience and consciousness

Consciousness is a state of mind characterised by an awareness of self and world. To offer a more detailed definition of consciousness would require that we deal with some very technical philosophical debates that ultimately are beyond the scope of this chapter, though it is worth noting that historically, the ideas of consciousness and conscience have been closely linked. Protestant teaching on conscience and Catholic notions of an examination of conscience were one factor that contributed to the focus on consciousness that characterises modern philosophy (Van Gulick 2014; Vendler 1989). The study of consciousness, in turn, has provided us with a more refined and nuanced understanding of the concept of conscience. Modern theories of consciousness inform the way in which we conceptualise the functions of conscience as a source of moral knowledge, moral motivation and moral reflection.

To address the issue under consideration, I would argue that conscience *requires* consciousness. Conscience, as we have defined it, is a mechanism that monitors the coherence between deeply held beliefs and practical action. But if we look more closely at conscience, we can provide a more precise specification of what this mechanism entails. Conscience is not an external observer that monitors the actions of agents. Rather, it is a constitutive feature of agency itself. That is, conscience involves a form of *self*-reflection. The Christian concept of examining one's conscience, for example, refers to an introspective activity whereby believers consider the extent to which they have lived in accord with God's commandments. An activity like this can only be carried out by agents on themselves. You alone have privileged epistemic access to all the relevant facts necessary to determine if you have acted rightly. Conscience, therefore, presupposes a capacity for self-reflection (or self-reflexive thought), and such a capacity is only had by conscious entities.

A critic might resist this conclusion and instead highlight the role that subconscious moral feelings play informing the moral actions of individual agents.

That is to say, we should not over-intellectualise the operations of conscience and require that agents have a second-order awareness of the operations of conscience. We might, for example, think of Mark Twain's novel *Huckleberry Finn*, where Huck, a 13- or 14-year-old white teenager, is travelling on a raft with Jim, an African American adult slave who has run away from his owner. Huck is emotionally torn about whether to turn Jim in or whether to assist him in his escape. Huck feels like he has a duty to turn Jim in, and indeed this sense of duty is described by Twain as originating from the boy's conscience, but Huck also has an intense, intuitive feeling of unease at dobbing Jim in and ends up refraining from exposing him (Twain 1884). This might seem to be the upshot of some subconscious process of moral reasoning rather than a fully conscious form of moral reflection. And so we might resist the idea that the activity of conscience only involves fully conscious processes of moral reflection. Conscience may also be said to have a subconscious dimension to it.

I am happy to concede that conscience can sometimes manifest itself in a subconscious feeling of unease rather than a fully conscious awareness of the moral character of an act. Yet I would still argue that consciousness is necessary even when we are dealing with the subconscious operations of the mind. Even subconscious feelings of unease or disquiet – such as Huck's feelings of emotional attachment to Jim – presuppose at least a limited degree of consciousness.

It is my contention that institutions do not have a conscience precisely because they lack consciousness. But an interlocutor might question this claim. Who is to say that institutions are not conscious entities? Could we not posit the existence of a collective consciousness had by institutions (particularly institutions that are well integrated)? The idea of collective consciousness, after all, is not a new one in the history of philosophy. Sociologist Emile Durkheim is sometimes interpreted as claiming that in some social situations individuals cease to be governed by their own beliefs and desires and rather have their behaviour determined by a collective consciousness acting through them. Durkheim (1898) uses the example of a person in a crowd who is carried away by mass emotion and cannot make any sense of what he or she felt after the crowd has disbanded. The claim is that in this situation the person's behaviour has been determined by a collective consciousness rather than individual desires and beliefs. In this sense, one could say that there are social situations where individual consciousness is subsumed into a form of collective awareness (Schweikard and Schmid 2013).

I do not wish to discuss the plausibility of the theory of collective consciousness that is attributed to Durkheim (though I would note that some theorists argue that Durkheim never held this view). I do, however, believe that the idea of institutional consciousness is implausible, as it ultimately goes far beyond what was ostensibly suggested by Durkheim. The claim appears to be that there is an additional consciousness over and above the consciousness of individuals. Yet it is not at all clear what this amounts to. It is unclear whether this collective consciousness has a bearing on the consciousness of individuals or whether it is completely distinct from the conscious experience of individuals. On the one hand, it would seem a stretch to say that individual behaviour is influenced by collective consciousness. Yet, on the other hand, if collective consciousness has nothing to do with individuals, then it would seem redundant as a means of explaining individual actions. It is controversial, therefore, to posit the existence of mysterious new phenomena in the social world – and theorists are understandably reluctant to do this (List and Pettit 2011, 4–5).

It could be argued that we need to posit the existence of group consciousness to explain the existence of joint intentionality in a group. By joint intentionality, we are referring to groups that jointly "intend" or seek to pursue a particular goal. Institutions, it could be argued, are made up of groups of people who jointly intend a particular goal or who are jointly committed to particular ideals. A Catholic hospital, for example, is made of individuals who are jointly committed to a particular healthcare mission, namely providing healthcare in the Catholic tradition (Tollefsen 2013). These individuals work together to realise a particular vision of healthcare and are motivated by certain religious institutional ideals. One might argue that some form of collective consciousness arises in such institutional contexts. Perhaps this might be conceived of in terms of a collective awareness among the staff. It could be argued that the staff are aware of each other and of the broader mission of the institution and that this is a kind of collective consciousness.

Yet the correct way to explain this phenomenon is to say that individuals are conscious of the collective rather than the collective itself possessing consciousness. That is to say, each individual member of the group has an awareness of being part of a collective; this should not be mistaken to mean that the collective itself is conscious. Furthermore, there are very plausible alternative psychological explanations available for the notion of joint intentionality – we need not appeal to an obscure notion of collective consciousness. List and Pettit (2011, 33) argue that groups have joint intentionality when they meet certain conditions, such as having a common awareness of a shared goal and having the intention of doing their allotted part in a more or less salient plan for achieving that goal. One need not posit the existence of group consciousness to claim that group intentionality exists. In the case of the Catholic hospital, it is sufficient to suppose that the staff involved have a shared goal and that they are acting with an awareness of the intention of others to pursue the same goal. We need not posit the existence of a level of consciousness additional to the consciousness of each individual involved.

If we are correct in denying that institutions are conscious entities, then this rules out the possibility of institutions having a conscience. Institutions lack the basic mental capacities necessary for conscious thought to exist (yet alone moral reflection). At best, institutions are groups of conscious individuals with certain shared goals and intentions. Yet this is a much more modest claim than suggesting that institutions are themselves conscious entities.

Institutions and the emotional sanction of conscience

So much for our discussion of conscience and institutional consciousness. As mentioned, my reservations are not confined to concerns about consciousness.

It also seems problematic to attribute conscience to institutions because they do not experience the emotional sanctions that are characteristic of the action of conscience. In what follows, I will refer back to the two hypothetical scenarios discussed in the section "The nature of conscience" and will consider what they tell us about institutions. My starting point in this discussion is that institutions do not experience emotions (at least not in any way similar to the way that individuals experience emotions). In light of this, I will use the analogy of the robot and the psychopathic doctor to show how institutions are unaffected when they act in a way that violates their basic beliefs. My aim is to show that institutions do not experience the emotional sanction of conscience as normal moral agents do.

In "The nature of conscience", I argued that the robot and the psychopathic doctor are not subject to the emotional sanction of conscience. If indeed the emotional sanction of conscience is absent from the experience of the robot and the psychopathic doctor, what might this tell us about institutions? It seems fair to say that institutions are like the robot and the psychopathic doctor insofar as they lack the moral awareness that we take to be characteristic of normal moral agents. The institution is like the robot insofar as it lacks consciousness. A robot may have the appearance of an entity that is consciously aware, but this is ultimately an illusion. Certainly, the robot does not have moral awareness in the sense of having a well-defined concept of right and wrong. It does not experience moral guilt when it fails to fulfil its function. Similarly, institutions are not conscious entities, as was shown in the previous section. Clearly, entities that are not conscious do not experience emotions. And so, just like the robot, institutions are not liable to moral distress if they are impeded from performing their function. Moral distress presupposes a capacity for a conscious, first-person experience of the world, and this is something that institutions lack.

Even if we were to assume that institutions have some degree of consciousness, this would not necessarily show that they experience moral emotions in the same way as normal moral agents. In the second scenario outlined earlier, the psychopathic doctor is consciously aware of the moral character of her behaviour, but she lacks an existential awareness of the implications of violating her conscience. She is unmoved by the voice of conscience, so to speak. The situation is similar with institutions. Even if institutions have some degree of collective awareness or intentionality, they do not have the same existential commitment to morality that an individual moral agent has. By an existential commitment to morality, I am referring to the awareness that individual moral agents have of their personal stake in living a moral life. For individual moral agents, living a moral life typically affects their character and identity in a very deep way (Fuss 1964; Bluestein 1993). Depending on how one lives the moral life, they are liable to be labelled a good or a bad person. Institutions, on the other hand, do not possess this awareness, at least not in any conscious way. On the contrary, institutions are more like the psychopathic doctor who lacks a conscious awareness of the moral implications of her actions. To be clear, I am not saying that institutions are immune from the negative impacts of departing from their own deeply held beliefs. But they certainly do not experience the psychological effects that make it emotionally costly to violate conscience. On the contrary, institutions lack the felt awareness of morality that is required to experience moral emotions.

Importantly, we need not focus just on morality. It may be that an agent is not particularly concerned about morality narrowly construed but is nevertheless invested in a series of ground projects (professional, familial and social) that in turn provide a source of meaning and purpose to their life. The agent in question would be liable to experience the emotional sanction of conscience should they act in a manner that somehow undermines or directly contravenes the commitments that characterise these ground projects. An institution, by contrast, would not be subject to emotional sanction should it depart from some aspect of its foundational ethos.

In light of this, institutions would not appear to experience the sanction of conscience in the same way as individual moral agents. Rather, institutions are better understood as corporate entities that at best experience the indirect effects of conscience through the conscious experience of their individual members.

One could make a functionalist objection to the arguments that I have just presented. Functionalism is the view that mental states are constituted solely by their functional role, namely their causal relations with other mental states, sensory inputs and behavioural outputs. One could argue that it does not matter what the material substrate is of the thing that we call conscience. Rather, one could argue that conscience is a functional property of things. That is, conscience is defined precisely by the way in which it makes it costly for an agent to act contrary to their deeply held beliefs. It is irrelevant whether an entity is actually conscious or not – what matters is whether the entity experiences the sanction of conscience in the form of distress and tension.

Yet this objection is unconvincing. It supposes that the existence of conscience is indicated by a functional property – namely the experience of some form of quasi-psychological tension, whatever that looks like – and not by the presence of a specific metaphysical property, such as a property of the brain. Institutions, however, do not even experience the psychological effects of the operations of conscience. Unlike individuals, hospitals cannot have or lose self-respect or a sense of dignity, and they cannot experience a loss of identity or moral integrity as a harm or injury. If we believe that moral distress is the functional characteristic of conscience, then we should not claim that institutions have a conscience. They do not experience moral distress in any meaningful way.

To be clear, I do not wish to deny that organisations are negatively affected when staff members act in a manner contrary to the institutional ethos. Indeed, I will explore this idea at length in Section 2 of this chapter. I do, however, think we need to be careful about defining conscience in terms of *anything* that is analogous to moral distress. Our definition may become so general that it would be very easy for anything to count as having a conscience. All it would take is the experience of disintegration as a result of an action that somehow violates core beliefs. According to this definition, we could say that a nation state has a conscience insofar as it experiences tension and disintegration when it violates certain core beliefs. Yet it seems a stretch to say that a nation state has a conscience in a literal sense.

In short, I do not believe that the functionalist account of conscience is strong enough to address the objections that people make to institutional conscience. Even if conscience were a functional property, part of the output of the conscience would still be the generation of negative emotions in response to wrongdoing. And you do not have this with institutions. The functionalist objection, therefore, would not be enough to salvage the idea of institutional conscience. This is not to downplay the impact of conscience-restrictions on individual members of institutions, which we will explore in the next section of this chapter.

Conclusion to Section 2

In this section, we have considered whether institutions can be said to have a conscience. I have presented two arguments that indicate that the answer is "no". I have argued that institutions do not have consciousness and therefore cannot be the bearers of a conscience. I have also argued that institutions do not experience the emotional sanctions that are characteristic of the work of conscience. In this respect, it is misguided to suggest that institutions have a conscience. It may be true to say that there is a "strong analogy" between individual conscience and institutional agency (Sulmasy 2008, 144). Yet this is a *very* different claim to arguing that institutions actually have a conscience. Equivocation on this issue in the literature is unhelpful.[4]

3. Does the question of conscience matter to the permissibility of institutional conscientious objection?

We have just considered whether institutions can be said to have a conscience. I have provided some reasons for thinking that this is incorrect. It remains to be shown, however, whether this question actually has bearing on the permissibility of institutional conscientious objection. Some theorists, in fact, characterise the question under consideration without any reference to conscience. Some theorists describe the question in terms of institutional non-participation, whereas others characterise the issue as one of religious liberty (Dickens and Cook 2000; Oderberg 2018; Shadd and Shadd 2019). The point is that we can talk about institutional liberties – like a hospital's right to "opt out" of the provision of medical procedures – without making reference to conscience.

In this section, I want to consider whether institutions could be said to have the right to conscientious objection independent of considerations pertaining to conscience. Specifically, I will examine whether one can make an argument by analogy from the conscience rights of individuals to the institutional liberties befitting healthcare providers. I will consider what criteria institutions must meet to ground a similar set of rights to those accorded to individual conscientious objectors. To be clear, this question differs from the question explored in Section 2, as I am not considering whether institutions literally have a conscience. Rather, I am exploring whether institutions may be deserving of a suite of rights analogous to the conscience rights that we accord to individual moral agents (what I have labelled *conscience rights**).

In the subsection titled "Institutions and the psychological costliness of violating core beliefs", I discuss whether institutions can be said to experience something analogous to the emotional sanction of conscience that might make them deserving of protection. I argue that it is only through its individual members that institutions are subject to the psychological sanction of conscience. The upshot of this, however, is that institutional liberties could be said to provide indirect protection for the consciences of individual healthcare professionals. In the subsection named "Institutional liberty as a means to protect individual conscience", therefore, I argue that conscience rights* for institutions are a means to protect individual liberty of conscience. In the subsection "Institutional integrity as a justification for conscience protections*", I make a separate argument for institution conscience rights. I argue that a loss of institutional integrity justifies the protection of institutional liberties in a manner analogous to individuals (cf. Bluestein 1993). Institutional integrity is a valuable property in and of itself in addition to being good for society.

Institutions and the psychological costliness of violating core beliefs

First, we should consider whether there is an analogy between the appeals to conscience made by individual healthcare practitioners and the claims made by healthcare providers seeking some sort of moral exemption. That is, we should consider whether there are analogous criteria that institutions meet that makes them deserving of something equivalent to conscience protections. As Wicclair (2011, 130) suggests, "claims can be advanced on behalf of hospitals that bear a family resemblance to appeals to conscience by individuals and warrant substantial deference". In what follows, I will consider whether healthcare organisations should be accorded conscience rights* on account of their moral similarity to individual conscientious objectors.

First, let us consider what analogous criteria institutions must meet to be deserving of conscience rights*. We might suppose that for institutions to be deserving of conscience protections, they must possess something equivalent to three traits we identified at the start of this chapter. First, institutions must possess the equivalent of deeply held beliefs. Second, institutions must have a mechanism for applying these "beliefs" to practical scenarios. Third, it must be costly for institutions to go against their deeply held beliefs. These traits are variants of the traits that we said that individuals must possess to be deserving of conscience protections (and, for that matter, to be ascribed a conscience in the first place). We should consider to what extent institutions can be said to possess something like these traits that justify a right to conscientious objection.

It seems fair to say that institutions have the equivalent of deep beliefs. As mentioned earlier, institutions have an identity and history that in many ways resembles that of individual agents. Institutions, like people, are in part defined by their core ethical commitments. Institutional values may be articulated in an institutional mission statement or an ethical code of conduct that the institution seeks to respect (O'Rourke 2001). Catholic healthcare providers in the United States, for example, seek to abide by the Ethical and Religious Directives for Catholic Health Services – an ethical code based on the teachings of the Roman Catholic Church (United States Conference of Catholic Bishops 2016). Alternatively, institutional values may be implicit in the history of an organisation. Many Catholic hospitals, for example, were started by religious orders, and these hospitals see the charism of their founding order as an important part of their institutional identity and mission. The value commitments and histories on which institutions model their practices are analogous to the basic ethical commitments and personal experiences that inform the practice of individual healthcare practitioners. Just as individual healthcare practitioners seek to practise in accord with their basic beliefs about morality and what is good for human beings, so do institutions seek to abide by an ethical code or mission statement that expresses their identity and history (Stempsey 2001, 3).

Institutions also have the mechanism for applying their mission statement to practical situations. Indeed, they express a kind of moral agency through the actions of staff who act in their capacity as employees and representatives of institutions (Bedford 2016, 261–262). Hospital administrators, for example, make decisions on behalf of the hospital about the treatments patients will receive, the services that staff will provide, and the strategic and research priorities that the institution as a whole will pursue. Healthcare practitioners, similarly, provide services to patients qua employees of the hospital. The institution acts through these individuals, at least insofar as these individuals have some official role in the organisation.

It is true that institutions do not literally perform medical interventions on patients. Institutions, furthermore, do not have a relationship with patients in the same way that a doctor or nurse does. Yet institutions are, nevertheless, deeply implicated in the actions of each of their staff members. A doctor who performs a sterilisation for a patient in a Catholic hospital, for example, is acting in their capacity as an employee of a particular institution. And the institution bears some responsibility for this action, even if the institution is not literally the agent performing the act (Sulmasy 2008, 143–144). Specifically, the action of an employee of an institution counts as an action of the institution, even if the action is not causally generated by the institution. As Shadd and Shadd observe, "health centres are constituted and animated by such people whose actions count as those of the institution" (2019, 971).

It is fair, therefore, to say that institutions have deeply held beliefs and that they also have a mechanism for putting these beliefs into effect. It is more difficult, however, to identify a specific psychological cost to institutions for deviating from their ethos. To refer back to the discussion in "Institutions and the emotional sanction of conscience", it is not obvious that there is a functional equivalent to the emotional sanctions experienced by individuals who violate their conscience. Institutions do not suffer the emotional sanction of conscience because they are not subject to strong emotions like individuals are. It does not seem that institutions are subject to moral distress in the same way as an individual (Wicclair 2011, 131). Institutions do not have to live with the haunting voice of conscience reminding them of the fact that they have acted in a manner contrary to their deeply held beliefs. They do not experience the pangs of guilt and shame in the same way that individuals do when they violate their conscience. Rather, institutions are inanimate entities, and they have no first-personal awareness of the world. If there is harm that institutions experience, it would be in the form of the experience of their individual members.

Certainly, the individuals who make up an institution can experience the psychological effects of conscience. Individual agents acting on behalf of institutions may still feel bound by their conscience to act in a morally upright manner. As such, they may be subject to the censure of their own consciences should they find themselves in an ethically compromising situation. We might, for example, think of the psychological burden that the members of an ethics board in hospital would bear if, say, they were pressured by external authorities into authorising a procedure that is directly contrary to the mission of the organisation. The members of the board may feel deep moral regret and compunction should they be forced to contravene the basic values of the institution. It is plausible to suggest, then, that there would be some instances when the members of an institution would experience serious psychological distress should they be required to violate their consciences.

Yet we are referring to individual members of the institution, not the institution itself. The individuals who make up an institution are not the same as the institution considered as a collective. And so we cannot just assume that the psychological distress of the individuals concerned carries over to the institution. One might, of course, argue that we can generalise our ascriptions of harm from individuals to institutions. Yet a critic might argue that it is double-counting to impute the harms experienced by individuals to institutions as well. If we are to attribute harm to institutions we would need to be able to identify a distinct harm that institutions experience over and above the harm experienced by individuals. There does not appear to be any psychological harm, however, that is additional to the harm experienced by individuals. Rather, it seems that we need to look at the moral integrity of an institution to locate the harm that an institution experiences when its members violate its mission and ethos. We will discuss this consideration in "Institutional integrity as a justification for conscience protections*". First, however, we will consider how institutional liberty provides a means by which to protect the conscience rights of individuals.

Institutional liberty as a means to protect individual conscience

Where does this leave us in assessing the permissibility of institutional conscientious objection? We have seen that institutions do not experience psychological distress in the same way that individuals do. In light of this, it would be wrong to base a right to institutional conscientious objection on the moral distress or moral injury that institutions stand to incur if they violate their basic beliefs. Institutional conscience rights*, however, are an important part of allowing healthcare practitioners to practise in accord with their conscience. Conscience rights* provide institutional protection for individual conscientious objectors who might in other institutional contexts be forced to violate their deeply held beliefs. As Wicclair writes,

> it can be important to physicians, nurses, pharmacists, and other personnel to be able to practice and work in a community that shares a commitment to a core set of goals, values, and principles.

> (2011, 131)

Even if we reject the claim that institutions experience moral distress, therefore, we still have reason to respect institutional independence simply because institutions are made up of individuals, and the consciences of those individuals matter. If we fail to respect institutional liberties, we may in fact be curtailing the rights of individuals to act in accord with their deeply held moral beliefs.

To better understand this argument, it is instructive to consider the example of a Catholic hospital. Many healthcare practitioners choose to work in Catholic hospitals as they feel that it is a professional environment in which they can still abide by their own deeply held moral values. Catholic hospitals have codes of conduct that rule out the performance of procedures that might challenge the moral code of a devout Christian or someone from another religious or ethical tradition who shares conservative Judeo-Christian values (United States Conference of Catholic Bishops 2018; Catholic Health Australia 2001). There is less risk of experiencing the moral distress that practice in a secular hospital might impose on someone who has a socially conservative moral code. The pressures to conform are far less pronounced when one is working in an institution that refuses to provide services such as abortion, gender affirmation treatments or euthanasia. As Wicclair writes,

> [p]racticing or working in an institution that permits actions that violate a healthcare professional's core values might compromise her moral integrity. At the very least, it can contribute to considerable moral distress.

> (2011, 131)

In sum, institutional conscience rights* can assist individual healthcare practitioners to practise in accord with their deeply held convictions.

An interlocutor might argue that the moral code of institutions can actually be harmful to individual conscience rights. It might be said that religious healthcare institutions that enforce a rigid moral code on their employees restrict their individual conscience rights rather than creating an environment where people can practise in accord with their beliefs. One might think that healthcare professionals deserve the right to exercise their individual professional discretion in their work. Wicclair, for example, argues that healthcare professionals should be given the positive right to object to laws or codes of conduct that prohibit particular morally contentious practices in medicine (Wicclair 2017, 16). Religious health-care providers' codes of conduct, however, prohibit individuals from providing services such as abortions or emergency contraception even where an individual feels bound in conscience to do so.

Yet, as Christopher Tollefsen has argued, this rejoinder misunderstands the nature of institutions and the values that they represent. An institution's values arguably represent the shared judgement of the group of practitioners who make up the institution. Tollefsen provides the example of Catholic healthcare institutions and their prohibition on abortion. He writes:

> Catholic health care professionals share a normative judgment that views unborn life as sacred and that involves a refusal to kill anyone, including an unborn child. Catholic institutions formed around a shared commitment to this norm thus prohibit direct abortion, and try, though perhaps not as hard as they should, to ensure that all who undertake the mission of the institution are on board with that institution's commitments regarding human life.
>
> (Tollefsen 2013, 239)

Not all Catholic healthcare practitioners would share the view that abortion is immoral, though Tollefsen is right to say that many Catholic doctors would hold this view. It is also fair to characterise Catholic healthcare institutions as coopera-tive endeavours whereby like-minded healthcare practitioners work together to realise a particular, religiously informed vision of healthcare.

Presuming this to be the case, we would actually undermine the religious lib-erty of a community of practitioners if we were to prevent them from enforcing a particular code of conduct within their institutions. That is to say, we would violate the consciences of many if we were to allow a few dissenting practitioners to practise in accord with an alternative and incompatible vision of healthcare. Tollefsen puts the point forcefully, arguing that

> [t]he idea of creating protections for positive rights of conscience for health care workers in Catholic (and many other religious) institutions, where the judgments of conscience in question run contrary to the foundational com-mitments of the institution . . . actually conceals a deeper antipathy to the rights of conscience and religious liberty that are exercised not just by indi-viduals acting in isolation from others, but by individuals acting coopera-tively together with others to serve essential goods in accordance with their deepest religious and professional convictions.
>
> (Tollefsen 2013, 239)

Accordingly, it would be wrongheaded to suggest that institutional conscience protections are somehow harmful to the conscience rights of individuals. Rather there is a sense in which we can see the code of conduct of institutions as a repre-sentation of the will of the individual members of the institution acting corporately for the sake of goals that can only be achieved through cooperation and mutual striving (cf. Bedford 2016, 261).

Tollefsen's argument becomes problematic, of course, when an insufficient portion of the staff population endorses or accepts the mission of the organisation. Yet assuming that the code is representative of the general will of the staff population, then it is deserving of respect. Here lies a deeper sense in which institutional liberties are related to individual conscience: institutional liberties facilitate a form of collective action whereby groups of practitioners are allowed to act together to realise a vision of healthcare to which they jointly subscribe.

Thus, institutional liberties play an important role in allowing individual healthcare practitioners to practise in accord with their values. It is my contention that this gives us a pro tanto reason for affording conscience rights* to institutions. To be clear, this argument would hold independently of what one thought of the importance of protecting so-called *institutional conscience*. We need not believe in institutional conscience to think that institutional liberties are worthy of protection.

Institutional integrity as a justification for conscience protections*

So far we have considered whether institutions experience moral distress in a manner analogous to individuals when they are forced to violate their conscience. I argued that institutions *do not* experience psychological distress but that institutional liberties are still worthy of protection on account of the moral distress that individual members of the institution might otherwise experience. I now wish to make a different argument for institutional conscience rights*. In this subsection, I will argue that there is an analogy between the loss of integrity experienced by individuals who violate their conscience and loss of integrity of institutions that violate their core beliefs and values. Both individuals *and* institutions experience a loss of integrity as a result of violating their core beliefs. And this gives us reason for granting conscience rights* to institutions. The harm to integrity may not necessarily be felt in the case of institutions, but it is a morally significant harm nonetheless.[5] I will first offer an account of why institutional integrity is of serious moral concern; I will then argue that we should afford conscience rights* to institutions to ensure that they are able to maintain their integrity.

According to one view – a view that I have developed in earlier chapters of this book – the costliness of violating conscience consists in a loss of integrity or a loss of coherence between one's actions and one's deeply held beliefs. A reader might wonder why it would be costly to lose coherence between one's actions and deep beliefs. One harmful effect is that an agent would undermine their own self-identity. Presumably, the constitution of the self involves processes of self-reflection and self-determination whereby an agent decides and consciously endorses a series of core beliefs about themselves and the world. If we abandon our self-identifying beliefs, however, we lose one of those features that helps to make us *a self*. We "undo" the self that we have fashioned over the years through our thoughts and actions.[6]

Deeply held beliefs and commitments are, of course, not the only constituent features of the self. If the self were nothing more than a series of beliefs and commitments, then agents who lacked deeply held beliefs would really have no grip on selfhood at all. Yet that seems implausible. But surely deeply held beliefs and commitments are a *very important* and *deep* part of the self, even if they are not the sole constituent feature. When one individual describes themselves to others, they will presumably describe a series of core commitments such as religious, familial, cultural and political commitments. Indeed, we need not be prescriptive about the kinds of commitments that an agent takes to be identity-conferring. What matters is that an agent has deep commitments, whatever these may be, and these commitments are seen to be a central part of one's moral character. Most agents would have certain deeply held beliefs that they take to be constitutive of their sense of self. When an agent gives up these deeply held beliefs, there is a very real sense in which the agent has a weaker grip on selfhood.

Building on this idea, we can offer a more precise specification of the impact that violations of conscience have on an agent. What they ultimately lead to is not so much as *loss of selfhood* as a *fracturing of the self*. If one does not act in accord with one's deeply held beliefs, a dichotomy arises between one's personal moral commitments and the way in which one interacts with others. One way to think about this is in terms of a split between one's *deep self* and one's *acting self* (Sripada 2016). We might think of the *deep self* as the seat of our basic, self-identifying moral beliefs, whereas the *acting self* is that aspect of our psychology that pertains to practical activity. The problem with violations of conscience is that they introduce tension between the deep self and the acting self. Rather than having our deeply held beliefs reflected in our actions, a conflict arises whereby our actions reflect a completely different set of commitments to the supposed constitution of our deep self. Our actions are a betrayal, so to speak, of the deep self.

Alternatively, we might conceptualise this conflict in terms of the *private self* and the *public self*. We might think of the *private self* as a person's privately held moral and religious beliefs, whereas the *public self* refers to the way in which one conducts oneself when acting in a public, professional capacity. As I suggested in Chapter 3, the self is fractured when the moral reasons that govern one's actions in private are distinct from the moral reasons that govern one's actions in the public realm (Atkins 2019, 472). Many proponents of political liberalism suggest that it is virtuous to set comprehensive doctrines aside when one is carrying out duties as part of public office (for example, when one is a lawmaker or a health bureaucrat) (Billingham 2017). This claim, however, overlooks the deep tension that is introduced in one's identity when one acts contrary to one's deeply held beliefs. When one behaves in public in a manner that is entirely contrary to one's own deep moral commitments, one undermines the unity of one's own identity. Rather than being a consistent individual, one comes to acquire multiple (and arguably incompatible) identities – a public persona that conforms to the standards of public morality and private identity that is shaped by one's considered beliefs about morality (MacIntyre 1999).

There are several other related reasons why we might see a loss of integrity as problematic. Some theorists argue that unity and the desire to repair "inner division" are admirable characteristics of persons, and, as such, violations of conscience and internal psychological discord are morally problematic (Bluestein 1993, 297). Bluestein suggests that we have a moral duty "to ourselves to lead personally integrated lives" and that in matters of inner unity, especially moral unity, our self-respect is at stake (1993, 297). Related to this, some theorists argue that unity or inner peace contributes to our having a good life (Benjamin 1995, 470; Bluestein 1993).

Yet it is unnecessary to explore the moral value of integrity in any further detail. I offered a detailed account of this in Chapter 3. It should suffice to note that integrity has significant intrinsic and instrumental value. In the remainder of this chapter, I will argue that there is an analogy between the harm incurred by individuals who violate their conscience and the harm experienced by institutions that are forced to violate their core commitments. Institutions, I would contend, experience a loss of integrity similar to individuals when they act in a manner contrary to their deeply held beliefs. In exploring this analogy, I will first discuss the core beliefs of institutions and the self-constitution of institutions before describing the harm associated with a loss of institutional integrity.

Institutions, like individuals, are defined by those core beliefs that characterise their mission. If we were to point to what makes one institution distinct from another, we would point among other things to the beliefs, intentions and aims that unite the individual members that make up each institution. As discussed earlier, religiously affiliated hospitals have a certain philosophy of care that informs the practice of healthcare practitioners who work in the hospital. The work of healthcare practitioners in Roman Catholic healthcare facilities, for example, will at least to some extent reflect Christian principles such as a respect for the dignity of persons and a desire to carry out the healing ministry of Jesus Christ (O'Rourke 2001; Taylor 2001). This may not necessarily lead to different practices, though sometimes it may. Catholic facilities may give more attention to services that are particularly central to their mission – such as care for people suffering from addictions and hospice care – whereas they may also refuse to provide certain services that conflict with their mission – such as euthanasia or surgical abortions (Wicclair 2011, 131–132).

It is tempting to view institutions in a static manner by focusing on the way that they appear to us in the present. There is, however, something analogous to a process of self-constitution that institutions undergo over time, and it is important that we be aware of this. The narrative of an institution is similar to a personal narrative (Linde 2009). Just as each person has a history, so too do institutions. Many healthcare institutions have existed for several decades if not centuries, and the events and experiences of the past inform the way in which the institution operates today (O'Rourke 2001, 15–16). There may be some degree of institutional memory that informs the way in which healthcare institutions practise today, and it is important that we are aware of this and the role that it plays in informing practice (O'Rourke 2001). The ethical standards of an institution will likely be reflective of many years of experiential knowledge as well as the foundational principles on which the institution is based (Hogan 2001, 163–165).

What might we say, then, of the impact of a loss of institutional integrity? I would argue that institutions sustain serious, morally significant harm when they are forced to violate their beliefs; importantly, this harm is experienced by those who form part of the institution as well as those who interact with the institution.

First, we should recognise that institutional integrity is valuable in and of itself. That is to say, it is better for an institution to be unified and morally consistent in its practices and activities rather than being morally inconsistent. There is a sense in which integrity is an admirable trait of institutions just as it is for individuals, and it befits institutions to seek to repair their integrity where this has been lost (Bluestein 1993, 297). Furthermore, one could argue that the existence of hospitals dedicated to upholding certain moral ideals is of intrinsic value to the society of which they form a part. As Wicclair (2011, 131) writes, "a society with hospitals whose identity is based in part on perceived moral ideals is a better society than one without such hospitals".[7] Where institutions are obliged to operate in a manner contrary to their core values, then, they stand to lose an intrinsically valuable trait. That is, the institution would be worse off *in se* if it were to lose or have diminished integrity.

A critic might argue that there is nothing intrinsically good about institutional integrity. An institution may be consistent and unified in its pursuit of evil ends, yet there does not seem to be anything admirable about such an institution. The Nazi Party may have been principled and consistent in its vicious persecution of minority groups in pre- and intra-bellum Germany; this does not make the integrity of the party an admirable trait. In saying that a person or an organisation acted with integrity, then, we fail to pass a clear and unambiguous moral judgement upon their actions. It would seem that our assessments of integrity would need to be combined with a moral assessment of the content of an institution's moral principles and actions. Self-standing attributions of integrity are morally incomplete (Audi and Murphy 2006, 11).

It is true to say that integrity in the pursuit of evil is not an admirable trait. If we presume, however, that an institution is pursuing morally good or at least morally neutral ends, it seems better in and of itself for the institution to pursue these ends in an integrated rather than a divided or disunified manner (Wicclair 2011, 131). The property of wholeness or wholeheartedness is a valuable trait for an individual or an organisation to have under normal circumstances – notwithstanding the concern that some organisations may have morally dubious aims. While my account of conscience in Chapter 3 focused more on the importance of moral purpose in an agent's life, I did not deny or negate the importance of moral integrity. On the contrary, moral integrity is part of what it means to have a sense of purpose in one's life. An agent who has purpose is an agent whose actions possess a coherence insofar as they are directed towards one particular aim.

Earlier we discussed the impact of a loss of integrity on the selfhood of moral agents. I argued that the self of moral agents can be weakened when agents abandon their deepest, self-identifying beliefs. This notion is helpful as a means to understand the intrinsic value of integrity for institutions. Integrity is a structural property that holds institutions together and helps them to survive. From the perspective of the institution and its own survival, surely it is valuable to have integrity and consistency. Without integrity, institutions would seem to face an existential threat. They would run the risk of *disintegrating* as a collective or group (Hogan 2001, 164–165). As evidence of this, we need only consider how integrity scandals in the corporate sector are often followed by the collapse of companies at the centre of such scandals (Petrick and Scherer 2003; Damiani, Bourne and Foo 2015).

Second, institutional integrity is a trait that has significant instrumental value. As Audi and Murphy observe (2006, 11), integrity is a trait "that is important for achieving overall moral uprightness", even if it is not itself a substantive feature of moral goodness. That is to say, integrity can plausibly be characterised as a formal property that assists an agent in living a moral upright life. It is a trait which helps agents form their own character and acquire virtues constitutive of a moral life. In the case of institutions, integrity is a property that assists an institution in acquiring those attributes that we take to be characteristic of ethical conduct at an organisational level (Audi and Murphy 2006). For an organisation to be ascribed virtues like honesty, transparency and beneficence, it must behave in a consistent manner across a variety of situations and for the right reasons. Integrity is a trait that is essential in this process, for it involves consistency and fidelity to core values. An organisation cannot be considered honest, transparent or beneficent if it is constantly acting in a manner contrary to its mission and values.

Building upon this, it should also be noted that integrity is of value for the realisation of the ends of the institution. Without some degree of unity of purpose, individuals who form part of a collective can be frustrated in their pursuit of certain goods that can only be realised collectively. If a Catholic hospital lacks a binding moral code, for example, it would impede the work of practitioners who want to realise a particular vision of healthcare (Iltis 2001). As Tollefsen observes, to prohibit the enforcement of an institution's code of conduct is to "deny the institution the liberty necessary to act socially for the sake of . . . shared [value] commitments" (2013, 238).

Finally, we should consider the impact that a loss of institutional integrity can have on members of the public who are reliant on these institutions. A loss of integrity may imperil an institution, and this may in turn have harmful effects on the public who rely on the institution for basic material, economic or social goods. In the case of healthcare institutions, if an institution is so deeply affected by an integrity scandal that it is forced to close some or all of its operations, this can have serious ramifications for the public and their ability to access healthcare (Sweeney and Geiger 2013). We should also consider that many religiously affiliated hospitals have a social mission and provide important social services to marginalised groups. As Wicclair suggests, "enabling Catholic hospitals to maintain a coherent identity and integrity benefits the community". He writes:

> If Catholic hospitals are not able to maintain their distinctive identity, they might decide to close their doors rather than compromise their integrity, which would leave more vulnerable members of the community worse off.

Moreover, in some communities, the closing of one healthcare facility can substantially reduce convenient access to health services for all residents.

(2011, 132)

In light of this, restrictions on institutional conscientious objection, which might be introduced under the banner of promoting the rights of vulnerable patients, may ironically have very negative effects on marginalised groups in the community. It is in the interests of the community that we support rather than undermine institutions seeking to practise in accord with a particular vision of healthcare.

Even if a loss of integrity does not destroy an institution, it may nevertheless lead to a trust deficit – something that recent experience has shown can easily arise when institutions fail to live up to their values. Members of society may no longer believe that healthcare institutions will provide services in a safe and timely manner. Healthcare institutions may be perceived as unreliable and untrustworthy as a result of repeated violations of their own moral principles. Indeed, this is arguably the situation that our society has found itself in, where there is a widespread suspicion of institutions and indeed widespread institutional breakdown (Gauchat 2012; Gawande 2016). We have an interest in allowing institutions to maintain their integrity insofar as this would be conducive to public trust in institutions.

In summary, this section has explored the impact that violations of conscience have on institutional integrity. I have argued that institutional integrity has significant intrinsic and instrumental value and that we have reason to respect an institution's mission and ethos if only to protect its integrity. Restrictions on institutional conscientious objection run the risk of undermining institutional integrity and may, in the process, undermine the very work of the institution and the services that it is supposed to provide. In light of this, there is, at least, a pro tanto case for respecting the right of healthcare institutions to opt out of participation in policies or practices that are contrary to their basic mission and values.

Conclusion

In this chapter, I have argued that institutions are deserving of conscience rights*, notwithstanding the moral and metaphysical differences between individual conscientious objectors and institutions. Section 1 of this chapter offered a brief account of the metaphysical nature of institutions. In Section 2, I argued that institutions do not have consciences. Institutions are not conscious entities, nor do they experience anything analogous to the emotional sanction of conscience. For this reason, it is misguided to claim that institutions possess a conscience. Section 3 of this chapter, however, argued that conscience is inessential to an institution's right to conscientious objection. I presented two arguments as to why an institutional right to conscientious objection should be respected irrespective of the existence of conscience. I argued that conscience rights* provide institutional protection for individual conscientious objectors who might in other institutional contexts be forced to violate their deeply held beliefs. I also argued that institutions will experience a loss of integrity if they are forced to violate their governing ethical principles. This in turn would have harmful consequences for both institutions and society.

There is an important question about what rights might compete with an institution's pro tanto right to conscientious objection. We might, for example, think of the right of consumers to access healthcare and whether this overrides an institution's right to conscientious objection (Schuklenk and Smalling 2017). Alternatively, it could be argued that the provision of emergency medical services is a more important goal than respect for institutional conscience (Wicclair 2018). As such, we may treat harm to institutions as a necessary evil to ensure that patients are able to access healthcare services in a timely and convenient fashion. This would mirror the argument with respect to individual conscience, namely that a patient's welfare should be a doctor's primary interest (Stahl and Emanuel 2017). One could argue that a similar principle applies to institutions.

I have not dealt in detail with the practical regulation of institutional conscientious objection, however, as this falls outside the ambit of the question under discussion in this book. My aim, rather, has been to show that there is philosophical case for conscience rights* independent of the notion of institutional conscience. In contrast to other authors (e.g. Sulmasy 2008; Bedford 2016), I have argued that institutions do not have consciences – not even in an analogous sense. Indeed, it seems that proponents of this stronger view confuse the notion of individuals exercising their conscience in an institutional context with the idea of institutional conscience. In my view, the language of institutional conscience may be a useful fiction to capture aspects of an institution's mission and the relationship that individuals have with institutions conceived of as a totality (Brown 2006, 416–417). Yet in the context of debates about conscientious objection, this fiction is a source of confusion rather than clarity.

These considerations notwithstanding, I have argued that we still have reason to respect the right of healthcare institutions to conscientious objection. Durland argues that "the very idea of institutional conscience as a freestanding structure sags atop buckling theoretical pillars" and that this gives us reason to "excise" institutional conscience protections from conscience legislation (2011, 1680, 1686). Yet I have presented arguments in favour of conscience rights* that do not depend for their validity on the idea of institutional conscience. Critics like Durland need to do more than critique the notion of institutional conscience if they are to make a compelling case against legislation such as the Church Amendments in U.S. federal law (Bertelsen 2013).

I believe that further scholarly research on the topic of institutional conscientious objection would be profitable both for ethicists and for policymakers charged with developing regulations surrounding religiously affiliated healthcare institutions. Approximately one in seven hospital patients in the United States are cared for in a Catholic facility (American Hospital Association 2018). This is to say nothing of the extensive healthcare services provided for patients by other, non-Catholic, religiously affiliated organisations. Evidently, policy questions surrounding institutional conscientious objection are of increasing relevance to the lives of ordinary citizens. It is my hope that this chapter may provide stimulus for detailed and nuanced reflection on the debate on these questions – something that has arguably been missing from public discourse to date.

Notes

1 In this section I do not purport to offer a strict metaphysical definition of the nature of an institution. Rather, I merely want to offer a rough account of the nature of healthcare institutions, with a view to considering what if any effects a loss of integrity might have institutions. For a detailed discussion of the metaphysics of institutions, including an exploration of how ideas from debates about personal identity might relate to institutional identity, see Rust 2019.
2 This scenario has been adapted from a thought experiment outlined in List and Pettit 2011, 19–20.
3 Later in this chapter, I will discuss the loss of integrity that comes from violations of deeply held beliefs and will consider how this affects individual moral agents as well as institutions. A loss of integrity is certainly part of the costliness of violating conscience and may be related to feelings of depersonalisation. Yet here I want to focus on the affective dimension of the phenomenon of depersonalisation.
4 Sulmasy (2008, 144) argues that "health care institutions have consciences, at least by a strong analogy if not also in fact". Yet this strikes me as a confused thought. For one, it is unclear what it means to say that institutions have "consciences . . . by a strong analogy". Either one has a conscience or one does not – conscience is not a property that is possessed in degrees or by virtue of a likeness to something else. Related to this, there is a major difference between saying that an entity has something *similar* to a conscience and claiming that an entity *has* a conscience. The kind of proof that one would have to offer for the latter claim is very different to what one would need to offer for the former claim.
5 By this I mean that institutions will not have a conscious experience of harm (as they are not conscious) but will be subject to harm nonetheless.
6 One could argue that we fashion a *new self* in the process, but then there would then be a question about whether this is indeed a positive change for an agent or whether something has been lost in the process of their change in identity.
7 A reader might take this quote to refer more to the instrumental value of institutional integrity rather than its intrinsic value. Yet if we presume that institutions are socially embedded institutions, then there is a real sense in which institutions form part of the fabric of society, and their value cannot be understood in isolation from the sociocultural matrix in which they exist.

References

American Hospital Association. *AHA Guide to the Health Care Field*. Washington, DC: American Hospital Association, 2018.

Atkins, Jed. "Integrity and conscience in medical ethics: A Ciceronian perspective". *Perspectives in Biology and Medicine* 62;3 (2019): 470–488.

Audi, Robert, and Murphy, Patrick E. "The many faces of integrity". *Business Ethics Quarterly* 16 (2006): 3–21.

Babbitt, Susan E. "Personal integrity, politics and moral imagination". In S. Brennan, T. Isaacs, and M. Milde (eds.). *A Question of Values: New Canadian Perspectives on Ethics and Political Philosophy*. Amsterdam & Atlanta: Rodopi, 1997: 107–131.

Bedford, Elliott Louis. "The reality of institutional conscience". *National Catholic Bioethics Center* 16;2 (2016): 255–272.

Benjamin, Martin. "Conscience". In W.T. Reich (ed.). *The Encyclopedia of Bioethics* (vol. 1.). Basingstoke: Macmillan, 1995: 469–472.

Bertelsen, Soledad. "Conscientious objection of health care providers: Lessons from the experience of the United States". *Notre Dame Journal of International and Comparative Law* 10;1 (2013): 122–148.

Billingham, Paul. "Can my religion influence my conception of justice? Political liberalism and the role of comprehensive doctrines". *Critical Review of International Social and Political Philosophy* 20;4 (2017): 402–424.

Bluestein, Jeffrey. "Doing what the patient orders: Maintaining integrity in the doctor-patient relationship". *Bioethics* 7;4 (1993): 289–314.

Brown, Grattan. "Institutional conscience and Catholic health care". In *Life and Learning XVI: Proceedings of the Sixteenth University Faculty for Life Conference*. Indianapolis: University Faculty for Life, 2006.

Catholic Health Australia. *Code of Ethical Standards for Catholic Health and Aged Care Services in Australia*. Canberra: Catholic Health Australia, 2001.

Childress, James. "Appeals to conscience". *Ethics* 89;4 (1979): 315–335; 328.

Cottingham, John. "Conscience, guilt, and shame". In Roger Crisp (ed.). *The Oxford Handbook of the History of Ethics*. London: Oxford University Press, 2009: 729–743.

Damiani, Claudio, Bourne, Naomi, and Foo, Martin. *The HIH Claims Support Scheme*. Canberra: Australian Government, 2015.

Dickens, B., and Cook, R. "The scope and limits of conscientious objection". *International Journal of Gynecology and Obstetrics* 71 (2000): 71–77.

Durkheim, Emile. "On social facts". In M. Martin and L. McIntyre (eds.). *Readings in the Philosophy of Social Science*. Cambridge, MA: MIT Press, 1994 [1898]: 433–440.

Durland, Spenser. "The case against institutional conscientious objection". *Notre Dame Law Review* 86;4 (2011): 1655–1686.

Frederick, Danny. "Pro tanto versus absolute rights". *The Philosophical Forum* 45;4 (2014): 375–394.

Fuss, Peter. "Conscience". *Ethics* 74;2 (1964): 111–120.

Gauchat, Gordon. "Politicization of science in the public sphere: A study of public trust in the United States, 1974 to 2010". *American Sociological Review* 77;2 (2012): 167–187.

Gawande, Atul. "The mistrust of science". *The New Yorker* 10th June 2016.

Hoffmann, Tobias. "Conscience and synderesis". In Brian Davies and Eleanore Stump (eds.). *The Oxford Handbook of Aquinas*. London: Oxford University Press, 2011: 255–264.

Hogan, Margaret Monahan. "Awaiting extinction or safe refuge in a culture of death". *Christian Bioethics* 7;1 (2001): 163–172.

Iltis, Ana Smith. "Organisational ethics and institutional integrity". *HEC Forum* 13 (2001): 317–328.

Linde, Charlotte. *Working the Past: Narrative and Institutional Memory*. London: Oxford University Press, 2009.

List, Christian, and Pettit, Phillip. *Group Agency: The Possibility, Design and Status of Corporate Agents*. London: Oxford University Press, 2011.

Lyons, William. "Conscience: An essay in moral psychology". 84;4 (2009): 477–494.

MacIntyre, Alistair. "Social structures and their threat to moral agency". *Philosophy* 74;289 (1999): 311–329.

McLeod, Carolyn. *Conscience in Reproductive Health Care: Prioritising Patient Interests*. New York: Oxford University Press, 2020.

Oderberg, David. *Opting Out: Conscience and Cooperation in a Pluralist Society*. London: Institute for Economic Affairs, 2018.

O'Rourke, Kevin. "Catholic hospitals and Catholic identity". *Christian Bioethics* 7;1 (2001): 15–28.

Petrick, Joseph, and Scherer, Robert. "Integrity capacity". *American Journal of Business* 18;1 (2003): 37–50.

Roberts, Tom. "Feeling nothing: Numbness and emotional absence". *European Journal of Philosophy* 27;1 (2019): 187–198.

Rust, Joshua. "Institutional identity". *Journal of Social Ontology* 5;1 (2019): 13–34.

Schuklenk, Udo, and Smalling, Ricardo. "Why medical professionals have no moral claim to conscientious objection accommodation in liberal democracies". *Journal of Medical Ethics* 43;4 (2017): 234–240.

Schweikard, David P., and Schmid, Hans Bernhard. "Collective intentionality". In Edward N. Zalta (ed.). *The Stanford Encyclopedia of Philosophy* (Summer 2013 ed.). Stanford: Stanford Metaphysics Lab. Available from https://plato.stanford.edu/archives/sum2013/entries/collective-intentionality/.

Shadd, Phillip, and Shadd, Joshua. "Institutional non-participation in assisted dying: Changing the conversation". *Bioethics* 31;1 (2019): 207–214.

Sripada, Chandra. "Self-expression: A deep self theory of moral responsibility". *Philosophical Studies* 173 (2016): 1302–1332.

Stahl, Ronit, and Emanuel, Ezekiel. "Physicians, not conscripts – conscientious objection in health care". *New England Journal of Medicine* 376 (2017): 1380–1385.

Stempsey, William. "Institutional identity and Roman Catholic hospitals". *Christian Bioethics* 7 (2001): 3–14.

Sulmasy, Daniel. "What is conscience and why is respect for it so important". *Theoretical Medicine and Bioethics* 29 (2008): 135–149; 138.

Sweeney, Anne, and Geiger, Kim. "Beleaguered Sacred Heart Hospital abruptly shuts". *Chicago Tribune* 7th July 2013.

Taylor, Carol. "Roman Catholic health care identity and mission: Does Jesus language matter?". *Christian Bioethics* 7;1 (2001): 29–47.

Tollefsen, Christopher. "Protecting positive claims of conscience for employees of religious institutions threatens religious liberty". *American Medical Association Journal of Ethics* 15;3 (2013): 236–239.

Twain, Mark. *The adventures of Huckleberry Finn*. London: Penguin, 2005 [1884].

United States Conference of Catholic Bishops. *Ethical and Religious Directives for Catholic Health Care Services* (6th ed.). Washington, DC: USCCB, 2016.

Van Gulick, R. "Consciousness". In E. N. Zalta (ed.). *The Stanford Encyclopedia of Philosophy*. Palo Alto: Stanford Metaphysics Lab, 2014. Available from: http://plato.stanford.edu/archives/spr2014/entries/consciousness/.

Velleman, David. *How We Get Along*. New York: Cambridge University Press, 2009.

Vendler, Zeno. "Descartes' exercises". *Canadian Journal of Philosophy* 19 (1989): 193–224.

Vujosevic, Marijana. "Conscience as the rational deficit of psychopaths". *Philosophical Psychology* 28;8 (2015): 1219–1240.

Wicclair, Mark. "Conscientious refusals by hospitals and emergency contraception". *Cambridge Quarterly of Healthcare Ethics* 20 (2011): 130–138.

Wicclair, Mark. "Conscientious objection in healthcare and moral integrity". *Cambridge Quarterly of Healthcare Ethics* 26;1 (2017): 7–17.

Wicclair, Mark. "Conscience clauses: Too much protection for providers, too little for patients". *American Journal of Bioethics* 18;7 (2018): 53–55.

Wood, Allen. *Kantian Ethics*. New York: Cambridge University Press, 2008: Ch. 3.

7 Conclusion

The role of conscience in medical practice and professional life

Introduction

This chapter summarises the content of the previous chapters and discusses the regulation of conscientious objection. I reiterate the need to adopt a more robust conception of conscience when thinking through the ethics of conscientious objection. I also discuss the importance of revising our understanding of medical practice. Commentators should cease to be preoccupied with service provision and ought to instead focus on the goods at which medicine aims. Once it is understood that conscience (and conscientious objection) is integral to medical practice, commentators and policymakers alike can more usefully direct their attention to ensuring access to services without attempting to suppress the exercise of freedom of conscience. I consider the implications of the framework presented in the previous chapters for the regulation of conscientious objection in medicine. I finish by discussing the broader relevance of a robust account of conscience for our understanding of ethics in professional life.

An appeal for consistency and reasonableness

It is apposite to begin this concluding chapter with an appeal for consistency and reasonableness in one's approach to the exercise of freedom of conscience in healthcare. It strikes me as odd that in liberal societies – where there is a presumption in favour of respecting the deeply held beliefs and convictions of moral agents – medicine has shifted in such a way that the deeply held beliefs and convictions of doctors are viewed with suspicion particularly where they have a manifestation within one's professional work as a healthcare practitioner. There seems to be fairly radical inconsistency in saying on the one hand that we ought to show deference for the lived experience and testimony of minority groups while claiming that doctors ought to suppress their own personal views about the goods of medicine and medical practice.

Indeed, multiple commentators in the bioethics literature adopt erroneous views on the issue of conscientious objection. Under the guise of defending liberal values, several commentators argue that we ought to introduce a near-total ban on conscientious objection. This has not always been the case. Yet in the past decade

DOI: 10.4324/9781003247623-7

academic bioethics has been characterised by a rather doctrinaire approach to the analysis of cultural and social issues in medicine. Rather than seeking points of compromise or consensus between rival viewpoints, academic bioethicists are wont to assert an absolutist position that gives little weight to the preferences of medical practitioners and instead prioritises patients and patient rights.

We ought also to be mindful that in much of society today there is a focus on what is often called epistemic injustice, an ethics and epistemology that focuses on injustices related to distrust and distortion of the testimony of certain individuals qua knowing subjects. Theorists of epistemic injustice argue that we ought to ensure respect for the testimony and "meaning making" of people in minority categories and ought not to exert power over their experience by attempting to redescribe their experience in terms that might be implicitly oppressive (Fricker 2007; Anderson 2020). The MeToo and BlackLivesMatter movements are both categorised by a concerted effort to lend credence to the testimony of disempowered persons – in one case women who have been the victims of sexual assault and in the other case blacks who are the victim of overt or systemic racism and police brutality. Judging by these social movements, it seems that there is an appetite in society to ensure that disempowered social groups are able to have their voices heard and receive justice.

The question in the mind of this author is why respect for the personal experience of moral agents is not extended to healthcare practitioners and physicians in particular. Granted, many argue that in the case of the doctor-patient relationship, patients are the disempowered party that we ought to focus on to ensure that power imbalances are redressed. There has, however, arguably been an overcorrection in medicine whereby patient rights have in some cases become the only ethical consideration deemed relevant whereas the interests of doctors (and their rights of conscience) have been deemed to be irrelevant. One author has gone as far as to argue that critics of conscientious objection are attempting to "bully" doctors into giving up their beliefs (Franklin 2016). It seems that we need to reconsider the expectation that doctors effectively abandon their own values when they enter clinical practice.[1]

It is my conviction that we ought to seek a reasoned middle ground on cultural issues in medicine and the issue of conscientious objection in particular. We ought to try to find solutions that give credence to the claims of both patients and clinicians and that seek to account for the valid insights of different stakeholders within the healthcare sector. In the context of the conscientious objection debate, this has sometimes been described as the compromise approach (though often what some theorists take to be a compromise might otherwise be construed as a near ban on conscientious objection) (Wicclair 2011). We should be wary of theorists who deliberately ignore or discredit views that fall short of suggesting a total ban on conscientious objection. Such an approach will not yield constructive and conciliatory solutions to disputes about the nature and scope of conscience protections in medicine.

Granted, some people may describe the views in this book as "strong" or "absolutist". I do assert the need to recognise that conscience is central to medical practice, so conscientious objection is unavoidable. Yet the problem lies not with my own viewpoint but rather with the assumptions implicit in recent literature on conscientious objection. Many of the assumptions on which the literature is predicated ought to be challenged.

Revising our understanding of conscience

Among other things, this book has sought to present a robust account of conscience and has argued that conscience ought to be recognised as a central feature of moral and professional life. I argued that conscience at the most basic level is concerned with a commitment to moral integrity and that restrictions on freedom of conscience prevent agents from living a moral life. I argued that conscience is a principle of moral awareness in rational agents and that it yields an awareness of the personal nature of moral obligation. I discussed the widely endorsed view that conscience monitors the coherence between an agent's self-identifying beliefs and intentions and their practical actions. I then considered how human beings are harmed when they are forced to violate their conscience. Restrictions on the exercise of conscience, I contended, undermine features of moral rationality that are a prerequisite of agency. One cannot act in a principled manner, either as a moral agent or as a medical professional, if one has no principles or if one's "principles" are received in an unreflective fashion or under duress from some external source.

Future moral philosophical scholarship ought to pay more attention to the indispensable role of conscience in professional life and more generally ought to acknowledge the serious impact that restrictions on conscience objection have on moral agents. To betray conscience is not just to forgo some desire or whim that one might otherwise indulge. Conscience is much more than a mere like or dislike. Conscience is a bedrock feature of the moral rationality of free agents. Without conscience, we have no principles, and without principles, we have no agency.

With this in view, theorists would do well to consider how we might integrate a notion of conscience into existing frameworks in moral psychology. Some moral philosophers, such as Velleman (2009) and Lyons (2009), have offered an overview of conscience drawing upon sources ranging from Freud and psychoanalytic theory to biblical accounts of anatomy. Philosophers of all traditions would do well to consider how a notion of conscience might be parsed by drawing upon the resources of their own philosophical schools. Conscience, after all, has a particularly diverse philosophical pedigree, and one's understanding of conscience can be greatly enriched by considering conscience's diverse historical and philosophical roots.

A more sophisticated account of conscience will help bioethical discourse move beyond the erroneous assumption that the exercise of conscience is foreign to medical practice. The moral calculus in the minds of many bioethicists is skewed greatly towards protecting the interests of patients, and this naturally leads one to suggest that conscientious objection ought to be heavily restricted if allowed at all. Yet we need to move beyond the idea of conscience as a set of arbitrary beliefs towards a view of conscience as constituting the core of the human person and an essential feature of one's ethical formation. Conscience is what in part defines an agent and her outlook on the world. There is a sense in which some very fundamental feature of moral agency disintegrates when an agent acts repeatedly in ways that are diametrically opposed to her personal belief system. They lose their own perspective on the world and become largely indistinguishable as moral agents as opposed to mere representatives of a received (but not interiorised) belief system.

A richer view of conscience will be the first step towards improving dialogue about the role of conscience in professional life. There are some theorists who extol the virtues of social conscience or physician activism on issues like racism while at the same time arguing for heavy restrictions on conscientious objection to abortion. I have made an appeal for consistency in one's thinking about social conscience and one's thinking about conscientious objection to socially contentious medical procedures such as abortion and euthanasia. We cannot expect physicians to compartmentalise their moral faculties in such a way that they suppress their considered views on some of the most fundamental social questions of our time.

My account of conscience also has implications for institutions that have a conscientious objection (as per my comments in Chapter 6). There is a sense in which an institution's mission and values are analogous to the fundamental commitments that characterise the life of an agent. The very raison d'être of institutions is articulated in documents such as a mission and values statements or an organisation's constitution. If an institution repeatedly acts in a manner contrary to their mission and values, however, the institution risks disintegration, or it may cease to resemble in any meaningful way what it was originally set up to be. At a time when social institutions are in crisis, governments ought to give serious consideration to the importance of institutional integrity if they are contemplating restrictions on institutional liberties. Undermining the integrity of institutions may only further exacerbate the deficit of trust that society has in institutions.

Revising our understanding of medical practice

In addition to revising our understanding of conscience, we ought to think seriously about assumptions implicit in contemporary understandings of medical practice. Consistent with the notion that conscience is integral to medical practice, much of my argument is concerned not just with how we understand conscience but also with the way in which we understand medicine as a social practice and as a professional discipline directed towards the goods of health and healing. Many theorists argue that medicine is a form of service provision and that doctors are in many cases *public servants*. I categorised this conception of medicine with the label *provider of services model of medicine* (PSM) (Curlin and Tollefsen 2021). Furthermore, doctors are sometimes described as fiduciaries of their patients who ought to always put patient preferences first in their decision-making.

Medicine, however, is best understood as a goal-directed practice that has as its object the goods of health and healing. The cultivation of character and virtue is essential to realising these goods of medicine, and part of this process involves giving physicians broad discretion to act in accord with their own considered understanding of good medical practice. We need to respect the discretionary space of physicians if they are to cultivate the sorts of virtues – integrity, fidelity and habits of moral reflection – that we take to be constitutive of excellence in professional life.

One might argue that the virtue ethical framework of medicine is too value laden to receive broad acceptance in a pluralistic society. But it is incoherent to praise pluralism and then refuse to accommodate plausible alternative views. The phenomenology of virtue, furthermore, is part of the fabric of the everyday experience of physicians. The importance of notions such as courage, integrity, consistency and moral reflection ought not to be controversial among physicians (otherwise one would wonder what else medical professionalism might conceivably consist in). Insofar as doctors want to be good doctors – doctors who practise the art of medicine with distinction – then they should be comfortable with an account of medicine that focuses on the goals of health and healing and the medical virtues requisite to realise these goods.

The regulation of conscientious objection

The discussion in this book has practical implications for how the state ought to accommodate the exercise of freedom of conscience in healthcare. I disagree with the prevailing views in the literature that conscientious objection ought to be heavily restricted if allowed at all. On the contrary, I think we need to give healthcare professionals a broad right to conscientious objection. Indeed, there should be a presumption in favour of conscientious objection in medicine provided that the practitioner(s) involved are expressing a viewpoint that has its origins in a fundamental life commitment and not just a mere dislike or distaste for a particular procedure. Given that the exercise of conscience (including objection) cannot be avoided, planning should include the development of mechanisms for addressing any problems that might arise from conflicts between the expectations/ demands of patients and the availability of services. But the onus should not be on conscientious objectors to have to justify their right to conscientious objection. In Chapter 5, I argued strongly against the idea of military-style tribunals for conscientious objectors.

I would challenge the view that conscience protections are going to have a catastrophic impact on service provision in healthcare or that it will lead to discrimination against certain categories of patients. Some critics of conscientious objection believe that increased protections for conscientious objectors could open the floodgates for irresponsible practices in medicine that will likely lead to significant numbers of patients missing out on access to basic medical care. Yet there is limited empirical evidence to support this conjecture (Roger and Blackshaw 2020). Particularly in light of the polemical tone of much of the literature on conscientious objection, it behoves critics to seek to evidence their claims that objecting physicians are creating serious and irremediable problems within the healthcare system (Harter 2021). At the very least there ought to be a well-evidenced case for the "burden" imposed by conscientious objection before we restrict what is one of the most fundamental rights of medical practitioners.

The same principles apply in the case of healthcare institutions. I have argued that institutions are deserving of a presumption in favour of the freedom to practise in accord with their mission and values. Institutional integrity is important for both institutions themselves and also society at large. We ought to respect institutional values, if only to ensure that institutions remain healthy and fully able to fulfil their indispensable social roles. There has been a concerted effort in the literature and in the popular media to provide evidence of the impact that restrictions on conscientious objection have on patients access to medical services – particularly emergency contraception and abortion (ACLU 2013; Nelson 2018). Institutional conscientious objection is said to prevent women in particular geographical locations from accessing contraception and abortion services in emergency situations. Yet I would argue that we need to view these accusations – while not negligible – in the context of the broader contribution that religiously affiliated institutions make to society in general and in particular to the well-being of society's most disadvantaged members. Religiously affiliated healthcare institutions perform an important social function, and we should be very wary of calls to force healthcare mandates on these institutions where they have an objection to the provision of particular procedures. Such mandates may lead these institutions to close their doors, which could in turn have very negative effects for society and particularly disadvantaged social groups. Yet even if we do not take into account the social mandate of these organisations, it remains the case that faith-based institutions are cooperative endeavours of groups of healthcare professionals working towards the goal of providing healthcare and healing for the general population. As such, we should in principle allow these groups to continue to operate in our pluralist society, granting that there will always be some degree of diversity and reasonable disagreement about the nature of health and healing.

Implications for the professions

It would be a pity if the implications of this book were taken to solely apply to conscientious objection. Much of what I had to say in this book is relevant to professional life in general and thinking through the moral psychology of professional ethics. We should not overlook the broader implications that a robust understanding of conscience might have for ethics in professional life. I have focused specifically on healthcare, though it strikes me that my argument could have implications for other flashpoints in the conscientious objection debate, such as law, education and hospitality. Conscience, after all, is a basic feature of human moral psychology and does not just come into play in the professional context of medicine.

One very simple example from the shipping industry might suffice to illustrate the broader relevance of the argument advanced in this book. For many decades, wharf workers around the world would on occasion refuse to unload cargo that they deemed to be morally objectionable in some way (Cole 2013). Wharf workers in San Francisco in the 1980s, for example, refused to unload cargo (mainly auto parts, steel and wine) from South Africa on account of concerns about racial inequality in that country. In another case, wharf workers in Durban in South Africa refused to unload ammunition and artillery cargo from a Chinese ship that was destined for Robert Mugabe's dictatorial regime in Zimbabwe. Wharf workers in both of these cases were concerned not to implicate themselves in the work of political regimes that they deemed to be objectionable.

One could argue that – on the same grounds that conscience ought to be respected in medicine – conscience, too, must be respected in the case of wharf workers who have a moral objection to participation in immoral practices such as commerce from racist regimes or the military supply of dictatorial regimes. While the employers of these individuals might argue that workers on the docks ought to set their personal morality to one side to ensure that reliable shipping lines are maintained, it could, nevertheless, be argued that the immorality of the kind of shipping concerned ought to be the pre-eminent moral consideration in this case. Or, more to the point, we ought to respect the deeply held convictions of the wharf workers in these instances, particularly seeing as their objection – far from being discriminatory – is, indeed, intended to militate against the actions of discriminatory and oppressive regimes.

If I were to express one particular hope for the impact of this book, it would be to prompt a new conversation about the role of conscience in working life. Professional and social ethics has, in many ways, come to largely ignore the moral psychology of practitioners and has instead focused on those who are in need of the services provided by the professions. It is high time that we shifted our focus towards the formation of virtuous professionals and considered how we can support this through the cultivation (rather than the suppression) of conscience.

Note

1 To be clear, I would not consider myself a "proponent" of standpoint epistemology, but I am simply making an appeal for intellectual consistency in the way in which we think about respect for the testimony and perspective of individual agents.

References

American Civil Liberties Union. *Miscarriage of Medicine: The Growth of Catholic Hospitals and the Threat to Reproductive Health Care*. New York: ACLU, 2013.

Anderson, Elizabeth. "Feminist epistemology and philosophy of science". In Edward N. Zalta (ed.). *The Stanford Encyclopedia of Philosophy* (Spring 2020 ed.). Available from https://plato.stanford.edu/archives/spr2020/entries/feminism-epistemology.

Cole, Peter. "No justice, no ships get loaded: Political boycotts on the San Francisco Bay and Durban waterfronts". *International Review of Social History* 58 (2013): 185–217.

Curlin, Farr, and Tollefsen, Christopher. *The Way of Medicine: Ethics and the Healing Profession*. South Bend: University of Notre Dame Press, 2021.

Franklin, James. "When the prescription is a lynching". *Quadrant Online* 21st September 2021. Available from https://quadrant.org.au/opinion/qed/2016/09/prescription-lynching/.

Fricker, Miranda. *Epistemic Injustice: Power and the Ethics of Knowing*. London: Oxford University Press, 2007.

Harter, Thomas. "Why tolerate conscientious objections in medicine?". *HEC Forum* 33 (2021): 175–188.

Lyons, William. "Conscience: An essay in moral psychology". *Philosophy* 84 (2009): 447–494.

Nelson, Lawrence. "Provider conscientious refusal of abortion, obstetrical emergencies, and criminal homicide law". *American Journal of Bioethics* 18 (2018): 43–50.

Roger, Daniel, and Blackshaw, Bruce. "Quotas: Enabling conscientious objection to coexist with abortion access". *Health Care Analysis* 29 (2020): 154–169.

Velleman, David. *How We Get Along*. New York: Cambridge University Press, 2009.

Wicclair, Mark. *Conscientious Objection in Health Care: An Ethical Analysis*. New York: Cambridge University Press, 2011.

Index

Entries in *italics* refer to figures.

For Product Safety Concerns and Information please contact our EU
representative GPSR@taylorandfrancis.com Taylor & Francis Verlag GmbH,
Kaufingerstraße 24, 80331 München, Germany

Printed and bound by CPI Group (UK) Ltd, Croydon, CR0 4YY
08/06/2025
01897008-0019